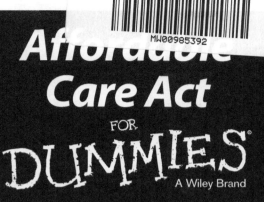

Affordable Care Act

FOR DUMMIES®

A Wiley Brand

Portable Edition

Affordable Care Act
FOR DUMMIES®
A Wiley Brand

Portable Edition

by
**Lisa Yagoda and Nicole Duritz,
with Joan Friedman**

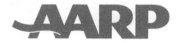

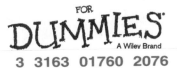

Affordable Care Act For Dummies,® Portable Edition

Published by
John Wiley & Sons, Inc.
111 River Street
Hoboken, NJ 07030-5774
www.wiley.com

For general information on our other products and services, please contact our Customer Care Department within the U.S. at 877-762-2974, outside the U.S. at 317-572-3993, or fax 317-572-4002. For technical support, please visit www.wiley.com/techsupport.

Wiley publishes in a variety of print and electronic formats and by print-on-demand. Some material included with standard print versions of this book may not be included in e-books or in print-on-demand. If this book refers to media such as a CD or DVD that is not included in the version you purchased, you may download this material at http://booksupport.wiley.com. For more information about Wiley products, visit www.wiley.com.

This and other AARP books are available in print and e-formats at AARP's online bookstore, www.aarp.org/bookstore, and through local and online bookstores.

Library of Congress Control Number: 2013958399

ISBN 978-1-118-86944-4 (pbk); ISBN 978-1-118-86939-0 (ebk); ISBN 978-1-118-86942-0 (ebk)

Manufactured in the United States of America

10 9 8 7 6 5 4 3 2

Contents at a Glance

Table of Contents

Introduction

● ●

*T*he federal Affordable Care Act (ACA), signed into law in 2010, is the most significant healthcare reform legislation since Medicare and Medicaid were established in the mid-1960s, and it's full of new benefits and rules being implemented over several years. We wrote this book to give you core information about what the ACA means for you and your family — how it can improve the quality of healthcare you and your family receive and what coverage options, benefits, and protections may be available to you. If you want to get the inside scoop on the basics of the ACA, you've come to the right place.

About This Book

You have a lot of choices for finding information about the ACA. You can visit AARP's easy-to-use online tool at HealthLawAnswers.org to get a customized report about the ACA and you, or you can visit AARP's HealthLawFacts. org or the federal government's www.HealthCare.gov site and many other online resources. You can tune into TV news programs and radio talk shows. You can read newspaper and magazine articles. Much information is being shared in every medium imaginable.

But if you're looking for ACA fundamentals all in one place, in a format that's user friendly and in language that's easy to understand, this is your go-to book. We want you to feel like you're getting the information from a friend who's well informed but not intimidating, as if you're sitting at the kitchen table talking about what the law is going to mean for you and your family.

We don't expect you to sit down and read this guide from cover to cover. Recognizing that your life circumstances are unique, we've designed this book so you can jump into a chapter or a specific section that's meaningful to you without having read what comes before. (If you can benefit from read-ing another part of the book, we let you know that.) You'll find information that's focused on helping you understand the law's impact, determine what (if anything) you may be required to do, and to give you step-by-step guidance so you can take appropriate action.

We also tell you where to look for answers to additional questions you may have.

A quick note to keep in mind: We include web addresses in this book, some of which may break across two lines of text. If you're reading this book in print and you want to visit one of these web pages, simply key in the web address exactly as it's noted in the text, as though the line break doesn't exist. (If you're reading this as an e-book, you've got it easy: Just click the web address to go directly to the web page.)

Foolish Assumptions

We wrote this book trying not to assume that you have any prior knowledge about what the ACA entails. We touch on all its key provisions to make sure you have a clear understanding of what to expect as you navigate the healthcare and insurance systems. Our goal is to provide the core facts about the ACA and not assume any prior knowledge.

We also don't assume that you lack health insurance coverage. In fact, given that nearly 85 percent of Americans do have some kind of coverage, we recognize that chances are good you may be one of them.

This book provides information for people with insurance, people without insurance, individuals, families, parents, parents-to-be, people with Medicare coverage, people with Medicaid coverage, small business owners, people who are unemployed, people who work part-time, people who work full-time . . . in other words, everyone! You may find that some sections, or chapters, don't apply directly to your situation, and that's fine; just skip them. Focus on what's relevant to your situation, and don't sweat the rest.

Icons Used in This Book

In the margins of this book, you'll see two graphical icons that help you home in on key points:

This icon sits next to paragraphs that contain information you want commit to memory — or at least revisit — to make sure you understand key impacts of the ACA.

This icon highlights helpful hints that can make it easier to benefit from ACA provisions or navigate the systems that have been set up to support the law.

Where to Go from Here

Honestly, that depends on you! We won't complain if you choose to flip the page (or scroll down on your e-reader screen) to start with Chapter 1 and read straight through to the end. But we recognize that you'll more likely use this book as a reference, and that's how we've created it.

Chapter 1 offers a nice overview of what the law does (and doesn't) do, but you may want to jump straight to Chapter 5 if you have Medicare and are concerned about how your coverage may be affected. If you're a small business owner, Chapter 7 may be your preferred first stop.

If you don't have any insurance right now and you don't know how to comply with the ACA, go to Chapters 2 and 3. If you're already insured and you're mostly curious about what the new law means for your existing coverage, Chapter 4 details the types of coverage that many insurers must provide under the ACA.

Use the table of contents to locate specific topics that are the most crucial to you. And don't forget to check out the book's Appendix, which lists more resources we highly recommend.

Wherever you go within the text, we hope you find the answers you need to reduce the worry or confusion you may feel about what the ACA means for you and the people you care about. And remember that you can always visit HealthLawAnswers. org for information specific to your situation.

Part I

Getting Started with the Affordable Care Act

getting started
with

the Affordable
Care Act

In this part . . .

✔ Get to know key consumer protections the ACA has put in place to help you improve your health coverage and avoid extravagant cost increases.

✔ Learn ways in which the healthcare law encourages preventive care, including for children.

✔ Discover who's exempt from needing to purchase a private insurance plan.

✔ Walk through the basics of the Health Insurance Marketplace (otherwise known as the *exchange*), including plan types, for people who need to shop for coverage.

✔ Identify essential benefits that every Marketplace plan must provide.

✔ Find out about income-based financial assistance available to people who shop on the Marketplace.

Chapter 1

The Nuts and Bolts of the Affordable Care Act

. . . .

In This Chapter

▶ Improving consumer protections

▶ Accessing new options for health coverage

▶ Getting more people insured

▶ Rolling out provisions step by step

. . . .

*O*ur focus in this book is to help you recognize how the Affordable Care Act improves the quality of healthcare you and your family receive. In this chapter, we introduce key ACA provisions. We start by outlining the consumer protections the ACA has established that benefit people who already have insurance as well as those who will purchase health insurance as a result of this legislation. We introduce the new way in which insurance is being sold: via the Health Insurance Marketplace. We also briefly explain what the ACA says about people who are uninsured and their options for securing insurance, how the law affects Medicare and Medicaid enrollees, and what the ACA means for businesses large and small. (These topics get more detailed coverage later in the book.)

Finally, we take a quick look at the timing of the ACA's key provisions so you have some insight into the legislation's impact from 2010 through today and into the future.

Improving Consumer Protections for Everyone

We want to start by outlining the consumer protections the law lays out.

Before the ACA, about 85 percent of people in the United States had healthcare coverage, whether through an employer plan, through a private insurance plan they bought directly, or through a government program such as Medicare or Medicaid. Although the ACA stands to have a major impact on the other 15 percent, the reality is that many of us won't be switching insurers or shopping for new plans because of the ACA. However, many of our current insurance plans will improve to abide by the law.

In the sections that follow, we explain the key consumer protections the ACA has established. Insurance companies must respond to these provisions by making sure their insurance policies — and companies' practices toward their customers — reflect this new reality. Employer plans must also make sure these protections are in place to keep healthcare coverage for their employees within the new law. So although the name of your insurance plan may stay the same, and you may not need to reenroll, chances are good that your insurer (or your employer) has updated your coverage because of the ACA.

Covering preexisting conditions

This provision is a big deal for people with diabetes, heart disease, a history of cancer, or any other serious health condition. In the past, if you were that person and you lost your insurance coverage (because the insurance company terminated your coverage, because you lost coverage from your job, or for any other reason), you likely faced an uphill battle trying to purchase a policy from another insurance company. When the company reviewed your application, your medical history was a red flag that may have sent you directly to the "coverage denied" pile.

As of January 1, 2014, all Americans are now eligible to purchase insurance, regardless of their health status or preexisting medical conditions. In other words, insurers may no longer deny coverage to anyone based solely on a preexisting health condition. Insurers also may not eliminate benefits, refuse to renew coverage, or impose a waiting period based on preexisting conditions.

Maintaining coverage during illness

For many years before the ACA's passage, a common practice among insurers seeking to deny payments for costly medical care was to reexamine customers' initial policy applications and cancel policies. Even if you purchased a health insurance policy, paid your premiums on time, and otherwise lived up to your end of the contract, an insurer could still find a way to drop your coverage if you became seriously ill or injured and your care threatened to become too expensive. When this happened, the insured paid the price — and sometimes literally went bankrupt as a result.

Under the ACA, as long as you pay your premiums, and as long as you were truthful when filling out your application paperwork, your health insurance is guaranteed. The healthcare law prohibits insurers from rescinding coverage because of unintentional mistakes or minor omissions on an application, and it prohibits canceling coverage based solely on your illness. So if you have coverage and you develop a condition that requires extensive treatment, as long as you live up to your end of the policy contract, your insurance company cannot cancel your coverage.

Regulating coverage and premiums to eliminate bias

Before the passage of the ACA, an insurance company could legally charge women more than men for the same policy. An insurer could also deny coverage to a woman based solely on gender. Companies made such decisions because women generally use more healthcare services than men. For example, to the insurer, a young woman might be considered a higher risk than a young man because she could incur substantial costs related to pregnancy.

Also before the ACA, an insurance company could — and often did — deny coverage to older people or charge them a significantly higher rate than a younger person for the same plan. (As we explain in a moment, insurers can still charge older people more, but the law sets limits.) And insurers frequently charged much higher rates or denied coverage to people based on their health status: If you had a history of illness, you could be denied coverage because of it or, at a minimum, you would pay more for your coverage than a healthier person.

The ACA has regulated these practices in two ways. First, the law states that an insurer must let you purchase a health policy regardless of your gender, health status, or similar factors that previously may have been used to predict how much you would use healthcare services.

Second, because of the ACA, insurance companies can take into account only four considerations when they set their policy premiums:

- **Age:** Although rates can still differ for older and younger adults, an older adult can be charged only up to three times more than a younger adult for the same plan. Three times may sound like a lot, but the legislation creates federal premium caps where none previously existed.

- **Geographic location:** Premiums are largely determined by where you live because of regional differences in the cost of medical care.

- **Tobacco use:** For the same policy, an insurance company can charge a tobacco user up to 50 percent more than someone who doesn't use tobacco. Some insurers have traditionally added a so-called "smoker surcharge" on premiums for tobacco users, who are more likely to develop long-term health problems than people who don't use tobacco. The ACA provision caps the premium difference for smokers while allowing a difference to exist as a deterrent to tobacco use — the largest preventable health danger in the United States.

- **Individual vs. family enrollment:** For obvious reasons, insurers still are allowed to charge more for a plan that covers your spouse and/or dependents than for a plan that covers only you.

As we explain in detail in Chapter 3, private healthcare plans sold on the Health Insurance Marketplace are available in five categories, per the ACA: bronze, silver, gold, platinum, and catastrophic. In each category, the insurance plan and the insured individual or family share costs differently: Some plans feature lower premiums and high out-of-pocket costs; other plans have the reverse.

When you shop for a plan on the Health Insurance Marketplace, you have the freedom to choose among these categories. In Chapter 3, we walk you through some key considerations when mulling over which category may be the best fit for your health and financial needs.

Removing coverage limits

Because of the ACA, an insurance company can no longer place lifetime dollar limits on your health coverage. In other words, insurers can no longer limit how much they will pay out in essential medical services over your lifetime. The ACA also bars insurance companies from imposing annual dollar limits on coverage. These provisions, which especially help people with serious diseases that require expensive treatment, are automatically in effect on all private insurance policies purchased or renewed after January 1, 2014. If you have a policy whose plan year starts in October, for example, then as of October 2014, you no longer are subject to these limits.

The ban on annual and lifetime limits applies to both employer-sponsored and individual plans, but only for the cost of what the law calls "essential health benefits." These benefits, which we outline in Chapter 3, are fairly broad and include emergency services, ambulatory patient services (which means outpatient care), preventive and wellness services, prescription drugs, maternity care, lab services, rehabilitative services, and more. However, be aware that certain types of treatments and costs may fall outside the scope of what the ACA deems essential health benefits. We encourage you to ask your insurer for examples of costs that aren't subject to this ban.

Certain health insurance plans qualify as being *grandfathered* and are not required to follow every aspect of the ACA as we're describing here. See the upcoming section "Recognizing exemptions for grandfathered plans" for the details.

Limiting out-of-pocket costs

Another significant financial protection the ACA provides relates to out-of-pocket costs. The maximum out-of-pocket costs for any insurance plan sold on the Health Insurance Marketplace (a topic we cover next) are $6,350 for an individual plan and $12,700 for a family plan. (The limits change each year to parallel increases in medical costs.)

Be sure to keep a couple of key points in mind about these maximums:

- The limits the ACA sets do *not* include your insurance plan premium, any balance-billed charges (money you may owe — especially when you get care outside of your plan's network — if a difference exists between what your provider charges and what your plan pays for that service), or costs for items that your plan doesn't cover. The SBC will set forth what's in this limit.

- Insurers count your copayments, coinsurance payments, and deductibles toward the out-of-pocket limit. Here's what these terms refer to:

  • *Copayment:* Your copayment is a fixed dollar amount that you pay out of pocket for a healthcare service (such as $25 for a visit to your primary care provider and $50 for a visit to a specialist).

  • *Coinsurance payment:* Some people think this term refers to a copayment, but it's a different out-of-pocket expense. A coinsurance payment is expressed as a percentage instead of a dollar amount. For example, your plan may require that you pay 20 percent of the allowed cost of a service. That 20 percent is your coinsurance payment.

  For example, say that your plan requires you to pay 20 percent of surgery costs up to a limit of $3,000. That means you're responsible for coinsurance payments (20 percent of the costs) up to $3,000 (after which the insurer pays 100 percent).

  • *Deductible:* Your deductible is the amount you pay out of pocket at the beginning of your insurance plan year before your insurance company pays toward your claims.

> ✔ If your household income falls below certain thresholds, insurers offering plans through the Health Insurance Marketplace must lower your out-of-pocket maximums for essential health benefits (which we detail in Chapter 3). We discuss these cost reductions in Chapter 4.

The out-of-pocket maximums reflect the most money you will pay during a given plan year (or during another set policy period) before the insurer has to start paying 100 percent of covered costs for your use of essential health benefits in the plan's network.

Noting other key protections

In addition to the items already covered, the ACA requires that insurance companies selling to individuals and small employers do the following:

> ✔ Fully cover certain preventive care services, such as cholesterol and blood pressure screenings, mammograms, colonoscopies, and recommended immunizations. Chapter 3 goes into more detail about what's considered a preventive service. For such services, you shouldn't pay a copayment or coinsurance payment, and you should get them free even if you haven't met your plan deductible. (Note, however, that you may encounter costs related to a service — for example, a facility or office fee — even if there is no cost to you for the screening test itself. And if the screening results in diagnostic services – for example, the doctor finds polyps during a routine colonoscopy – you may be charged for their removal and biopsy.)
>
> However, if you have coverage through a large group plan or if your insurance plan is grandfathered, you may not get this preventive coverage. See the next section for an explanation of grandfathered plans.
>
> ✔ Allow you to select your doctor (and your children's doctor) from your plan's provider network.
>
> ✔ Allow you to seek care from an OB-GYN without a referral from your primary care provider.
>
> ✔ Let you get care from an out-of-network emergency room service without paying a higher copayment or coinsurance

payment than you'd pay in network. (This way, you don't have to pay higher costs for getting emergency care out-of-network if you're away from home and need emergency care. But the out-of-network provider may still be able to bill you if the amount your plan pays is less than its charges.

✔ Provide coverage on a parent's family plan for adult children under age 26, even if they are married, not living with their parents, eligible to enroll in a plan at work, or financially independent. Note: Employers are not required to offer family plans. Check with your employer first to see if it does.

This provision aims to reduce the number of uninsured young adults and ease parental worries. In the past, young people were typically forced off their family's health plan upon turning 18 or 21 or when graduating from college.

✔ Share publicly its reasons for raising your premiums more than 10 percent, and get approval for doing so from the state insurance commissioner. This protection is called *rate review.*

✔ Spend at least 80 percent of the premiums they collect to pay for healthcare and quality improvement. Only 20 percent (or less) of premiums collected should be spent on a company's administrative, marketing, and overhead costs. If the company doesn't hit this ratio in a plan year, it could possibly owe its customers a rebate for a portion of the premiums they paid. This rebate may come in the form of a rebate check, a lump sum deposit to the account you used to pay the premium, or a reduction on future premiums. If the rebate goes to your employer, your employer can pass it along in any of these same ways or use it to improve your coverage.

✔ Give you a Summary of Benefits and Coverage (SBC), which is a document that spells out your benefits and coverage in language that is easy to understand. All SBCs must follow a standard outline (see Chapter 2 for an explanation). That way, if you're shopping for insurance coverage, you can look at two or more SBCs and do an apples-to-apples comparison.

If you're already insured and your insurance company hasn't yet given you an SBC for your current plan, call or e-mail the company to ask for one. If you have an employer-sponsored plan, ask your human resources department or benefits administrator for the SBC. You can also request a glossary that companies must provide to help explain healthcare and medical terms.

✔ Offer you the right to appeal its decisions, such as the denial of a claim. In its paperwork noting such a decision, the insurer must explain why it denied the claim and explain your right to appeal. If you request that the company reconsider such a decision, your insurer must do so. If the decision stands, you have the right to request a review by an independent organization that then determines whether to accept or overturn the insurer's decision.

Recognizing exemptions for grandfathered plans

Certain types of insurance plans are considered *grandfathered* and, therefore, are subject to only some of the ACA's provisions, not all of them. What defines a grandfathered plan is quite specific.

A grandfathered plan refers to individual and employer plans that were in existence by the day the ACA was signed into law (March 23, 2010) and have stayed basically the same since that date. You may have enrolled in your employer plan *after* that date, but if the plan existed and has stayed basically the same since March 23, 2010, it may be a grandfathered plan. If you enrolled in a plan sold in the individual market after that date, your plan isn't grandfathered.

The first item to know is that your insurance company or employer must inform you if you have a grandfathered plan. In the information you receive explaining plan benefits, the insurer or employer must state whether a plan is grandfathered; you shouldn't have to do any guesswork.

Over time, plans that are currently grandfathered may change coverage to remain competitive and profitable; they would then lose that grandfathered status and need to comply with the ACA.

If your plan *is* grandfathered, here's what you need to keep in mind:

- As with all insurance plans, the grandfathered plan must adhere to these ACA provisions:

  - It cannot place a lifetime limit on coverage.

  - It cannot terminate someone's insurance coverage unless that person has purposely given false information when applying or has neglected to pay the premiums.

  - It must allow adult children up to age 26 to get coverage under a parent's family insurance plan.

  - It must provide a Summary of Benefits and Coverage to its existing customers.

  - It must spend at least 80 percent of the premiums it collects on healthcare costs or quality improvements (instead of on overhead, administrative costs, or marketing).

- Unlike other private insurance plans, a grandfathered plan *isn't* required to do the following (although it may do so voluntarily to provide better service and compete more effectively with other plans):

  - Cover the essential health benefits required by the ACA, which we outline in Chapter 3

  - Allow you to choose your own doctor from within its network of providers

  - Let you use an out-of-network emergency room without paying more than you would for in-network care

  - Limit your out-of-pocket expenses

  - Set premium levels based only on the criteria outlined in the earlier section "Regulating coverage and premiums to eliminate bias"

  - Grant you the right to appeal its decisions, such as the denial of a claim

  - Publicly state why its premiums are increasing by 10 percent or more

- Also, if you have an *individual* grandfathered plan — one that you purchased yourself, not through your workplace — that plan may still have annual limits on coverage and may be able to deny coverage for preexisting conditions.

If you have a private individual insurance plan that you bought for yourself or your family, definitely find out whether it's grandfathered. If it is, you may want to at least do some comparison shopping on the Health Insurance Marketplace in your state. (We introduce the Marketplace in the next section.) Your grandfathered plan is required to give you a Summary of Benefits and Coverage (SBC), which makes it fairly easy to compare what you've got with other plans that are available to purchase.

Establishing the Health Insurance Marketplace

As part of the healthcare law, every state has a Health Insurance Marketplace, also referred to as an *exchange,* where people looking for coverage can go online to shop for health insurance. Some states created their own Health Insurance Marketplace; where states have not done so, the federal government administers the Marketplace. Think of the Marketplace as an online shopping mall for health insurance that makes it easier to find health plans in your state and choose one that works well for you.

The Marketplace is a new way for people to shop for health coverage. If you enroll in the Marketplace, it also determines whether you are eligible for health coverage through a public health program such as Medicaid.

Keep in mind that you don't *have* to shop for insurance coverage on your state's Marketplace website. You can still purchase coverage elsewhere — from an agent, broker, or online insurance company, for example. **However, if you want help to lower your costs based on your income, the only place to do so is the Marketplace**. Every plan offered on a state's Marketplace site is a *qualified health plan,* which means it has been vetted to make sure it complies with ACA requirements for benefits, costs, and so on. Note that you may use the Marketplace only until you are eligible for Medicare. The Marketplace is primarily for people under age 65 who need insurance. Generally, if you're 65 or over and you apply to the Marketplace, you'll be directed to enroll in Medicare.

Here's another key consideration: You can't enroll in a Marketplace plan anytime you want. If you experience what's called a *qualifying life event,* such as losing your job, getting divorced or married, or having a baby, you're granted a special 60-day Marketplace enrollment period during which you can shop for a plan on the Marketplace. Otherwise, you must wait for an open enrollment period. Open enrollment for the Marketplace lasts for about two months each year. To secure coverage for 2015, for example, the Marketplace open enrollment period is slated to start on November 15, 2014, and to end on January 15, 2015.

Interacting with your state's Health Insurance Marketplace involves these steps:

1. **Connecting:** You can go to the Health Insurance Marketplace website for your state and view the available plans. To find the Marketplace website for your state, you can start at www.healthcare.gov/ what-is-the-marketplace-in-my-state or www.HealthLawAnswers.org.

   On your state's Marketplace website, you set up an account (see Chapter 2) and will learn whether you are eligible for financial help and can review each plan that offers what you need. You find out its costs — including what the premium will be if you qualify for financial help — and see what's covered so that you can make an informed decision about which plan to purchase.

   If you don't use a computer, you can shop the Marketplace by phone at 800-318-2596 or find someone to speak to in your local area by going to LocalHelp. HealthCare.gov and typing in your city and state or zip code.

   For more ways to connect, including using the chat function and getting non-English support, see "Getting Marketplace help" in Chapter 2.

2. **Comparing:** Your state's Marketplace lists all plans in one place and provides a Summary of Benefits and Coverage (SBC) using a standardized form that the ACA requires. That way, you can make side-by-side comparisons of the benefits and prices; you're comparing apples to apples. The ACA requires that an SBC

describe what's included in a plan in simple language, so you should face very little guesswork about what's covered.

Every Marketplace plan is required to cover essential health benefits, including doctor visits, hospital care, emergency care, prescriptions, preventive care, and more (see Chapter 3). Differences among plans relate to what's covered beyond those essential benefits, provider networks, and how you and the plan share expenses. (If you want to pay a lower premium, for example, you may be looking at a higher deductible if you use your health coverage for something other than preventive services.)

3. **Choosing:** After you've reviewed your options, you can choose the health plan that works for you and sign up.

The ACA has established for the first time financial help to pay for health insurance. Some people who buy a plan in the Marketplace get help covering the costs. Low-cost plans are also available, depending on your income. For example, a family of four earning less than $94,200 a year may be able to get financial help.

If you want help preparing yourself for a positive interaction with your state's website, turn to Chapter 2 for a detailed explanation of how to do what you need in the Marketplace. Refer to Chapter 4 for information on how you can save money when you purchase insurance through the Marketplace.

Covering More People

The U.S. Department of Health and Human Services developed five goals for the ACA and multiple objectives to support each goal. For example, the first goal is "Strengthen Health Care," and here are three of that goal's supporting objectives:

- ✔ Make coverage more secure for those who have insurance, and extend affordable coverage to the uninsured

- ✔ Improve healthcare quality and patient safety

- ✔ Emphasize primary and preventive care linked with community prevention services

In the following sections, we discuss the impacts the ACA has on individuals and families, on people who qualify for Medicare and Medicaid, and on businesses.

What the ACA means for individuals and families

The first section of this chapter, which outlines consumer protections of the ACA, provides a good overview of the law's key provisions that benefit almost all individuals and their families. These protections aim to reduce unexpected health-care costs, address waste and fraud in the healthcare system, and improve the quality of care people receive. A long-term result should be a healthier America, gained one person and one family at a time.

The consumer protections are a big part of the ACA picture. Another major part is what individuals and families are required to do to comply with new rules under the ACA.

Unless you are a member of an exempted group (as discussed in Chapter 4), you must have health insurance coverage as of 2014. To use terminology you've probably heard in news stories, you must adhere to or satisfy the *individual mandate*. If you can afford insurance but choose not to enroll in a plan (assuming you don't already have coverage), you face two types of financial costs:

- **You're assessed a fee.** You pay the higher of these two amounts:

  - A percent of your annual household income. (We explain the cap on how high this amount can be in Chapter 4.)

  - A flat rate (fees assessed monthly for the months you don't have insurance)

  As we explain in Chapter 4, this fee will increase every year, and to encourage compliance with the ACA, it is being phased in over three years, starting in 2014.

- **You have to pay for your medical care.** One impetus of the ACA is to make sure the cost of healthcare is shared among as many people as possible. In the past, uninsured people may have gotten medical treatment but failed to pay for it. When they received uncompensated care, other people (such as employers and insurance customers) footed the bill in the form of higher premiums. Now, if you don't carry insurance and you need care, you will have to pay out-of-pocket and may rack up medical debt that for some may lead to bankruptcy.

Keep in mind that you don't have to purchase an individual, private health insurance plan (whether through the Marketplace or otherwise) to meet the individual requirement to have insurance. You also meet the requirement if you are insured by Medicare or Medicaid (which we discuss next), if your child is covered by a state Children's Health Insurance Program (CHIP), if you participate in a group plan through an employer, if you have coverage through the military or a veterans' program, if you have a grandfathered individual plan, or if you have other health insurance coverage that is sufficient.

What the ACA means for people who have Medicare

We hear a lot of questions and concerns from Americans who have Medicare. We have good news: The ACA *does* have some impact on people covered by Medicare, and the impact is quite positive.

The ACA protects the guaranteed Medicare benefits you were promised. The law also adds more services for people who have Medicare; reduces prescription drug costs; and adds new resources to fight fraud, scams, and waste, helping the Medicare program save money.

Under the ACA, people who have Medicare Part B are eligible for the preventive and wellness benefits that include an annual wellness visit, immunizations, mammograms, and other screenings for certain diseases, including diabetes and certain cancers. For instance, Medicare Part B wellness visits allow people to update their personalized prevention plan with their doctor every year. You no longer pay a copay or deductible amount when you have this type of care.

The change in preventive and wellness benefits for people with Medicare stands to help a lot of people. In 2011 alone (the year after the ACA was passed into law), more than

32.5 million Americans in traditional Medicare used one or more of the program's free preventive services, and more than 1 million people took advantage of the new annual wellness visit.

In addition, people with Medicare Part D now receive discounts on prescription drugs while in the coverage gap known as the *doughnut hole.* This term refers to a gap in prescription coverage that starts after your Medicare plan has paid a certain amount of money for medications during a plan year and ends after you've reached your yearly limit in out-of-pocket costs.

Under the ACA, people with Medicare Part D who fall into the prescription drug coverage gap receive more than a 50 percent discount on many brand-name prescriptions in 2014, as well as a discount on generic drugs. Since the law's enactment, millions of people with Medicare have saved billions of dollars on prescription drugs. In 2012, Part D enrollees who reached the doughnut hole saved an average of $706 a year in their prescription costs. Under the ACA, the Part D discounts will gradually increase until 2020, when the doughnut hole will effectively be closed.

We devote Chapter 5 to a more complete discussion of how the ACA and Medicare intersect. If you currently have Medicare or will soon be eligible to enroll, we encourage you to check out that chapter.

What the ACA means for the Medicaid program

Medicaid is a health coverage program for individuals and families with low income, as well as some older people, pregnant women, and people with disabilities. Under the ACA, states have the option of expanding Medicaid eligibility so that it can include millions more people than it did before the ACA's passage.

A key Medicaid-related provision sets a uniform income eligibility level that applies throughout the country. States that agree to extend Medicaid coverage to adults under age 65 who earn up to 138 percent of the federal poverty level receive federal funding supporting that expansion. To ease states' financial burden for enrolling new people in Medicaid, the federal government is footing the bill for three years starting in 2014 and will continue to pay the bulk of the associated costs for new eligible adults after the first three years.

The result of these changes is that some people who were previously not eligible for enrollment in Medicaid may be able to get coverage through this program as of 2014. Anyone who enrolls in Medicaid has met the requirement to have health insurance and doesn't need to purchase any additional insurance coverage.

Now for the tricky part: When the Supreme Court ruled in June 2013 on the constitutionality of the ACA, it determined that the law cannot force states to expand Medicaid. Instead, each state may make its own decision regarding whether to expand the program. Some states have opted to expand Medicaid, and others have opted not to. States that have chosen not to may alter that decision in the future. Therefore, people wanting to secure Medicaid benefits must find out the laws in their own state.

People who earn too much money to qualify for Medicaid in their state, but who have children and need low-cost access to healthcare coverage for them, can still apply for the Children's Health Insurance Program (CHIP) in their state. Every state offers CHIP coverage, although that coverage differs from state to state. In some states, parents and pregnant women can enroll in CHIP, as well. The ACA provides for funding for CHIP for several years. In addition, in states that opt to participate in Medicaid expansion, the ACA enables some children and families previously covered by CHIP to transition to Medicaid. But CHIP remains intact and funded, and additional ACA provisions are encouraging more streamlined systems to help low-income families find the coverage they need among Medicaid, CHIP, and the Health Insurance Marketplace.

What the ACA means for businesses

The ACA's impact on businesses differs depending on their size. The ACA doesn't affect more than 95 percent of U.S. businesses because they have fewer than 50 full-time equivalent employees. But the small percentage of U.S. businesses that have 50 or more full-time equivalent employees are required to provide insurance coverage that meets established minimum standards or face a potential tax penalty. The requirement generally applies to firms with 100 or more full-time equivalent employees starting in 2015 and employers with 50 or more full-time employees starting in 2016.

The two key criteria here are the affordability of the coverage the business offers and the minimum value of that coverage:

- ✓ **Affordability:** For employee-only coverage (meaning not for a family policy), the employee's share of the lowest-cost plan's premium costs cannot be more than 9.5 percent of that person's annual household income. If the cost of the lowest-cost coverage the business provides is higher than that percentage, the plan is considered not to be affordable.

- ✓ **Minimum value:** The company's health coverage must pay for at least 60 percent of the costs of covered services to qualify as having minimum value under the ACA.

A larger business that doesn't provide coverage meeting these two criteria may face a financial penalty called an *Employer Shared Responsibility Payment* as of 2015. This payment is calculated based on whether the company offers any insurance coverage to its employees. If the company doesn't offer any insurance, each year it will owe $2,000 per full-time employee, excluding the first 30 employees. If the company does offer insurance, but the coverage is found lacking per one or both criteria, each year it will owe $3,000 per full-time employee who receives financial help for a plan through the Health Insurance Marketplace.

These penalties are designed to encourage larger business to take responsibility for providing adequate coverage to employees, reducing the number of uninsured workers in the country and improving access to healthcare.

But what about smaller businesses that employ fewer than 50 people? Will they face the same tax penalties as their larger counterparts for not supplying coverage to their employees?

The answer is no; the ACA doesn't require small businesses to offer insurance to their employees. However, the law changes for the better how a small business can shop for health coverage. If you're a business owner with 50 or fewer employees, you can now join with other small businesses in your state to get health insurance for your employees. For the first time, you should have many of the same options that previously were available only to larger companies.

Business owners can shop for health insurance plans for employees using their state's Health Insurance Marketplace. Within each Marketplace is a Small Business Health Options Program (SHOP) that facilitates comparison among plans, including benefits and costs. Owners can choose what plan to offer to employees, and then those employees can go and sign up through the SHOP Marketplace. The system is designed to reduce a business owner's paperwork and administrative costs, in addition to providing greater leverage for driving down costs by grouping coverage purchases for many small businesses.

In addition, small businesses purchasing coverage via SHOP may be eligible for a tax credit to help make the cost of covering employees more affordable. For a more detailed discussion of how the ACA impacts businesses and their employees, turn to Chapter 6.

Implementing the Timeline for Key ACA Provisions

We realize you may not be interested in a history lesson; your focus likely is on figuring out what the ACA means for your life and how to navigate provisions that apply to you. However, as more people become aware of the ACA and realize that it's changing the way healthcare functions in this country, it seems worth offering a quick overview of when key provisions were established and what additional measures will come into play in the future. Here's the rundown of how the ACA has played out so far and what you can expect going forward:

2010

Individual and small group health plans must cover more preventive care than they did previously. Health screenings and tests for certain cancers, diabetes, and heart disease are covered if they're recommended for you.

Health plans can't drop your coverage if you get sick.

Health plans cover children on your family plan up to age 26.

Health plans can't put dollar limits on how much they'll pay for covered benefits over your lifetime and must start phasing out annual dollar limits on your covered benefits.

Children up to age 19 can't be turned down for health coverage because of a preexisting condition.

Small businesses with low-wage workers can qualify for a tax credit for up to 35 percent of their cost for health coverage.

2011

Medicare covers more preventive care health screenings and tests than it did previously.

The Medicare Part D prescription drug doughnut hole begins to close. The discount in 2011 is 50 percent for brand-name drugs and 7 percent for generic drugs.

Health plans have a limit on how much of premium revenue they can devote to profits and administrative costs compared to what they spend on patient care.

2012

The Medicare Part D prescription drug doughnut hole continues to close. The discount in 2012 is 50 percent for brand-name drugs and 14 percent for generic drugs.

2013

The Medicare Part D prescription drug doughnut hole continues to close. The discount in 2013 is 52.5 percent for brand-name drugs and 21 percent for generic drugs.

The Health Insurance Marketplace opens, allowing people to compare health plans, get questions answered, and enroll in plans for coverage that begin in 2014.

2014

The Medicare Part D prescription drug doughnut hole continues to close. The discount in 2014 is 52.5 percent for brand-name drugs and 28 percent for generic drugs.

Individuals, families, and small businesses have new ways to shop for coverage in the Health Insurance Marketplaces.

Financial help is available through the marketplaces to pay for coverage for low- and moderate-income families.

Health plans can't charge you more based on your health history or gender.

Health plans must cover the costs of approved clinical trials.

States have the option to expand their Medicaid program to cover more people with limited incomes.

No one can be denied coverage just because of a preexisting condition.

Most people must get health coverage or pay a tax penalty.

The small business tax credit increases to cover up to 50 percent of the employer's cost of coverage bought through the Health Insurance Marketplace.

2015

Larger businesses (employing the equivalent of 50 or more full-time people) must provide employee insurance coverage that meets established minimum standards or face paying penalties.

2015–2020

The Medicare Part D prescription drug discounts in the doughnut hole increase incrementally until it is effectively closed in 2020.

Chapter 2

Navigating the Health Insurance Marketplace

*T*he Health Insurance Marketplace, established under the ACA, is a new way for individuals and small businesses to compare insurance plan options available in their state and buy insurance. Insurance companies compete for customers, and comparing prices is easy. (In a few states, however, there may be only one company selling plans.)

In this chapter, we walk you through the key information you need to know about the Marketplace so you can feel more comfortable going online and interacting with it. We start by explaining who needs to enroll on the Marketplace (versus who may simply want to stop by to compare prices or visit out of curiosity). We then note how you can shop for individual plans offered in your state, why comparing plan costs and coverage should be straightforward, and what you can expect when you apply for coverage.

 If you're a small business owner or manager, be sure to check out Chapter 7, where we explain the Small Business Health Options Program (SHOP), which allows you to compare plans that you may want to offer to your employees.

Determining Whether You Need to Enroll

How can you determine whether you should enroll through the Marketplace? Here are answers to some common questions:

 ✓ **Will I have to buy my health insurance through my state's Health Insurance Marketplace?**

   If you already have health coverage that meets a minimum standard, you don't have to enroll in a Marketplace plan. You don't need to use the Marketplace if you're among the vast majority of Americans who get their insurance through an employer or through Medicare, Medicaid, TRICARE (which offers insurance to active members of the military), the Veterans Administration, or another government program. If you get employer early retiree health benefits, you're already covered as well and don't need to shop on the Marketplace (although if you do, you may qualify for financial help).

 ✓ **Who will use the Marketplace?**

   You'll likely use the Health Insurance Marketplace if you're uninsured or need to buy coverage on your own because you don't have access to health insurance through an employer or other source such as Medicare or Medicaid. Members of Congress and their staffs also will buy their health insurance through the site.

 ✓ **Can anyone else shop on the Marketplace if they want to?**

   Yes. If you now buy your own insurance on your own, you can use the Marketplace.

   You may also use the Marketplace if you can't afford the lowest-cost plan that your employer offers. Your employer's plan is considered affordable under the ACA if your premium for an individual policy (as opposed to a family policy) for the lowest cost plan your employer offers amounts to less than 9.5 percent of your annual household income. If the percentage is higher than 9.5, or if your employer's plan doesn't offer *minimum value* (meaning it pays for at least 60 percent of the costs of covered healthcare services), you can shop for a replacement plan on the Marketplace.

To be clear, almost *any* individual may shop for a plan on the Marketplace during the Marketplace open enrollment period (which we explain in the upcoming section "Understanding enrollment periods"). However, if you're currently enrolled in an employer's plan that is deemed affordable and provides at least minimum value to you, you cannot qualify for financial help that other individuals may qualify for based on their household size and income. So the premiums you may pay on the Marketplace may be different from the premiums paid by people who qualify for financial help through premium tax credits.

✔ **If I'm uninsured, can't I shop for a plan somewhere else?**

Yes. Nobody is forced to use the Marketplace to buy health insurance. Individuals can still deal directly with insurance companies or brokers, if they choose.

However, one purpose of the Marketplace is to help the uninsured be able to afford to buy insurance. In addition to requiring that the Marketplace serve as a one-stop shop where people can compare and buy insurance coverage from a number of companies, the ACA requires that the Marketplace help people who struggle to afford insurance find financial assistance. Federal government subsidies to help pay for insurance (which we explain in Chapter 4) will be available *only* to individuals who purchase their policies through the Marketplace.

By applying for coverage through the Marketplace, consumers can find out whether they qualify for a tax credit to help pay for their insurance — which is up-front financial help to immediately lower the cost of premiums — or whether they qualify for Medicaid, the federal–state health program for low-income people (refer to Chapter 1).

✔ **How much financial assistance can I get to help pay for insurance?**

When you apply for health insurance through the Marketplace (a process we outline later in this chapter), you find out whether you qualify for help with your monthly premiums, out-of-pocket expenses, or both. The answers depend on your household size, annual household income, and whether you're eligible for other coverage.

For example, in 2014, individuals with income up to $45,960 and couples with income up to $62,040 may qualify for financial assistance. People who qualify can have the new tax credits sent directly to the insurance company.

✔ **As a single person, what if I earn $50,000 a year and my employer doesn't offer insurance? Do I qualify for financial help in the Marketplace?**

Most likely not. As a single person earning that amount, your income puts you over the limit for help as of 2014 unless you have deductions that take you below the threshold. (Income thresholds will change over time to reflect cost of living increases.) You are responsible for paying all your premium costs.

✔ **If I work for a small business that doesn't offer its employees health insurance, do the owners have to do so now? Or do I need to use the Marketplace to find a plan?**

Small businesses — ones with fewer than 50 full-time-equivalent workers — don't have to offer insurance. They've never been required to do so, and the ACA doesn't change that requirement. If your employer doesn't offer insurance, you can shop for an individual policy on the Marketplace, where you may qualify for help in paying your premiums.

✔ **I have cancer, and my wife has diabetes and high blood pressure. Can we get insurance through the Marketplace?**

Yes. Even if you've been turned down before, you can use the Marketplace to buy coverage. Nearly half of Americans age 55 to 64 have a preexisting condition that in the past could lead to denial of coverage. As of 2014, insurance companies are prohibited from denying coverage solely because of preexisting conditions (refer to Chapter 1).

Some *grandfathered* individual plans (those that aren't subject to all the ACA's provisions — see more about this in Chapter 1), which someone buys directly (not through an employer), may maintain coverage restrictions even under the ACA. If you have such a plan and you develop a medical condition it doesn't cover, you can use the Marketplace to switch plans.

✔ **I'm turning 65 this year. Can I use the Marketplace if I want to?**

You may use the Marketplace only until you are eligible for Medicare. The Marketplace is primarily for people under age 65 who need insurance. If you're 65 or over and you apply to the Marketplace, you'll be directed to enroll in Medicare.

If you currently have Medicare, you don't need to buy insurance through the Marketplace. If you turn 65 and enroll in Medicare, you'll no longer require insurance coverage from another source to be legal under the ACA. Turn to Chapter 5 for a discussion of how the ACA does and doesn't impact Medicare.

✔ **I lost my job and now work part-time. My employer doesn't offer insurance for part-timers. Can I use the Marketplace?**

Yes, and depending on your income you may qualify for financial aid if you buy health insurance through the Marketplace. For example, a single, 61-year-old nonsmoker making $35,000 is eligible for a subsidy on the Marketplace and would pay about $277 a month in premiums for the midlevel silver plan.

✔ **My employer offers insurance, but I can't afford to pay for my husband's coverage. Can I use the Marketplace?**

Financial assistance depends on whether the government considers your employer's plan affordable. To qualify, your employer's lowest-cost plan must require you to pay more than 9.5 percent of your total household income for your own coverage, not family coverage. You can also use the Marketplace and possibly get financial assistance if your employer's plan doesn't meet certain minimum standards and doesn't pay at least 60 percent of your expected healthcare costs.

For example, if your total household income is $80,000, the cost of your own employee coverage must be more than $7,600 annually to get help with paying for your premiums.

✔ **Compared with what I've paid in the past for individual coverage, will I pay more or less for insurance when I buy through my state's Marketplace?**

It depends. You have to do your own research (starting with checking your options on the Marketplace) to find out for certain. Plan prices can vary widely from state to state, and Marketplace options will change over time, as well.

Keep in mind that insurers are permitted to charge higher rates for older people — though less than what many companies charged older people before the ACA — and may charge smokers a 50 percent premium surcharge (refer to Chapter 1).

For all these reasons, the answer to this question very much depends on your specific circumstances.

✔ **What happens if I don't buy any kind of health insurance and remain uninsured?**

You may have to pay a tax penalty on your federal income tax. The ACA gives religious groups opposed to accepting insurance benefits, Indian tribes, and people whose household income is below the threshold for filing a tax return, among others, an exemption from penalties.

The phased-in penalty for not having insurance in tax year 2014 is $95 per adult or 1 percent of income, whichever is more, and for a family, the higher of $285 or 1 percent of family income. See Chapter 4 for more details about the financial consequences of not seeking coverage.

Under the ACA, you won't incur a tax penalty if you're uninsured for short periods of time; if you have a break in coverage of less than three months, you won't face a penalty.

Searching for Plans in Your State

First things first: Although the Health Insurance Marketplace is an online shopping platform, the federal government recognizes that not every American has access to a computer. If you don't use a computer, you can shop the Marketplace by talking to someone by phone at 800-318-2596. In every state, trained navigators provide personal assistance. (Foreign language assistance is available in 150 languages.) If you prefer to shop for plans outside the Marketplace, you also can shop with the help of licensed insurance agents and brokers.

If you do have computer access, the way to start shopping for a plan is to locate your state Marketplace site. Begin by going to www.healthcare.gov/what-is-the-Marketplace-in-my-state or www.healthlawanswers.org and then search for your state in the drop-down list.

Note that, before you can begin shopping, you may have to set up an account on your state's Marketplace. That process is fairly simple, and we explain it in the upcoming section "Getting Signed Up."

Private insurance plans

Shopping for a private insurance plan — meaning one an insurance company offers (instead of the government) — should be more straightforward than in the past, for a couple key reasons:

✔ All plans sold in the Marketplace are required to offer the same set of essential health insurance benefits, which we detail in Chapter 3. These benefits include doctor visits, emergency services, lab services, hospital stays, preventive services, prescription drugs, mental healthcare, newborn and pediatric care, and more. Before a plan is offered on the Marketplace, it goes through a vetting process to make sure it adheres to the ACA's requirements for benefits, costs, and so on.

✔ All Marketplace plans must provide a Summary of Benefits and Coverage (SBC) using a standardized form that the ACA requires. The SBCs allow you to make side-by-side comparisons of different plans' benefits and prices. An SBC must explain what's included in a plan in simple language, to eliminate confusion and guesswork about what's covered.

Given that all plans on the Marketplace must at least offer the same essential health benefits, can you expect that all the plans offered in your state will cost about the same amount? No. Here are the key reasons for cost differences among plans:

- ✔ **Various cost structures are available.** As you discover in Chapter 3, you can choose from four levels of coverage: bronze, silver, gold, and platinum. (You also may be able to purchase a catastrophic plan.) Each plan has different premium costs and out-of-pocket costs (including deductibles and copays). The bronze plans have the least expensive premiums but the highest out-of-pocket percentages. A platinum plan is at the other end of the spectrum, offering the lowest percentage of out-of-pocket expenses in exchange for the highest premiums.

- ✔ **You can select among plans that offer broader or narrower access to healthcare providers.** For example, you may buy into a *Health Maintenance Organization* (HMO), which operates in a local area and may provide coverage only if you go to the doctors and hospitals within the plan's provider network. Or you could select a *Preferred Provider Organization* (PPO) plan that has a provider network but also covers you if you go to doctors and hospitals outside the network. Broader access to providers (as with a PPO) costs more than restricted access to providers (as with an HMO).

- ✔ **Coverage still differs among plans.** Even though you're guaranteed that a Marketplace plan will cover the essential health benefits as identified by the ACA, not all plans cover them the same way or cover the same items beyond those essentials. If you have a history of requiring certain types of care based on a chronic condition, be sure to study each plan (and ask questions of a Marketplace customer service representative or navigator) to determine whether a given plan covers your specific healthcare needs.

Some state Marketplaces are more robust than others. If you live in an area with a large population, chances are good that multiple private plans may work for you, and you need to spend some time doing apples-to-apples comparisons (which the SBCs make easy) to figure out your best option. In other areas, you may find that only one or two plans fit your needs, so your shopping experience may mostly involve determining what to expect from the coverage being offered.

Either way, don't expect that you'll hop on your state's Marketplace website and spend 5 minutes exploring your options and enrolling. You're making a major purchase, and you need to devote some time to understanding what you're getting and what you'll pay. We recommend setting aside an hour *at the minimum* to look at plans, compare your options, and enroll. The more time you spend up front making a decision, the better that decision is likely to be.

Medicaid and CHIP plans

First, a couple quick definitions:

- ✔ **Medicaid:** The Medicaid program provides health insurance coverage for low-income individuals and families, as well as for some older people, pregnant women, and people with disabilities. Each state runs a Medicaid program, but those programs can differ from state to state in eligibility requirements and benefits.

- ✔ **CHIP:** The Children's Health Insurance Program is also offered in every state but differs among states. This program covers people who earn too much money to qualify for Medicaid but who have children and need low-cost access to healthcare coverage for them. (In some states, CHIP covers parents and pregnant women, as well.)

The ACA raised the income threshold for enrolling in Medicaid so that millions more people qualified for this program. However, the Supreme Court struck down the law's provision making Medicaid's expansion mandatory in all states. As a result, each state is making its own decision whether to participate in the expansion or stick with its previous income limits for enrollment.

For anyone uncertain about Medicaid or CHIP qualification, the Health Insurance Marketplace is streamlining the process of determining eligibility for these programs and getting enrolled. Some states' Marketplace websites offer direct links to Medicaid enrollment, for example. In all cases, your state's Marketplace can help you determine whether you qualify for Medicaid or CHIP.

If you're uninsured and have low income, don't risk incurring a tax penalty for not having any health insurance — although if your income is too low to pay taxes, you won't incur a penalty. Visit your state's healthcare Marketplace, or www. healthlawanswers.org, as soon as possible to find out whether you qualify for Medicaid, CHIP, or financial assistance with purchasing a private plan.

Comparing Coverage and Costs

When choosing a health plan, be sure to consider and compare the major factors of a plan's coverage and cost to make sure you know how it works and how it would work for you. Each has its own unique set of questions. By considering each of these factors, you can choose the plan that works for you and your family.

Coverage

Coverage refers to the range of health services your plan covers, such as doctor visits, hospital visits, maternity care, emergency room care, and prescription drugs. In Chapter 9, we outline ten essential benefits provided by the ACA. You want to see what the plan offers, whether it has limits on types of services, and how often you can use them in a year. You can start to understand your coverage using your Summary of Benefits and Coverage. Here's how:

- ✔ **Find out if the plan limits which doctors, hospitals, and other providers you can use.** Is your favorite doctor part of the network? What happens if you want to see an out-of-network provider? Will you have to pay more? Are the in-network doctors and hospitals conveniently located for you?

- ✔ **If you spend a lot of time out of state, check to see if you can get healthcare services in other states.** Also determine what the provider network looks like outside your home state or whether care will be out of network.

- ✔ **Find out which services are excluded from the plan.** If you know you will need a specific type of care — for example, bariatric surgery — you want to make sure the plan offers that type of coverage.

- ✔ **Check out the prescription drug coverage.** Make sure the plan covers the prescription drugs you take regularly and find out whether it requires any pre-authorization and works with a pharmacy in your area. See if you can receive your prescriptions by mail.

Cost

Be sure to understand the costs of your coverage:

- **Premiums** are the regular monthly payments you pay to your plan.

- The **deductible** is the amount you have to pay for health services each year before the plan covers costs. Say you have a $1000 deductible. You will have to pay $1,000 out-of-pocket for covered services before your plan will cover any costs. Once you've paid this amount, you've satisfied the deductible for the rest of the calendar year. Some services you can get without having to pay a deductible, such as preventive care.

- **Coinsurance** or **copayment** is a portion of the cost you may have to pay when you go to the doctor, get a prescription, or use other covered care.

  - *Coinsurance* is a percentage amount, such as 20 percent of the allowed cost of a doctor visit.

  - A *copayment* (or *copay*) is a set dollar amount. For example, you may pay $15 for each prescription or doctor's visit.

  Note: Prescription drugs may have copayments for some drugs and coinsurance for others.

- **Out-of-network providers** are doctors or other health professionals who are not part of your plan. Check to see if you have to pay more for an out-of-network provider.

  Keep in mind that plans don't have to count what you spend for using an out-of-network provider toward reaching your annual out-of-pocket limit (which we explain in Chapter 1). Out-of-network providers may also bill you for any difference between what your plan pays them and their charges.

We can't tell you what your insurance premiums and out-of-pocket costs will be, but we can offer a general guideline that may help as you start the process of searching for coverage: If you qualify for financial help on the Marketplace (meaning that you're currently uninsured, you have an individual plan now, or your employer's plan isn't deemed sufficient per the ACA requirements), you can expect to pay between 2 and 9.5 percent of your income to purchase a plan. The span reflects the fact that your income level determines the amount of financial assistance available to you. The Marketplace offers the greatest financial help to those at the lower end of the income scale.

Plus, as we note earlier in the chapter, many low-income people are finding that they qualify for Medicaid in their state.

How to compare

When it comes to comparing plans on your state's Health Insurance Marketplace, the Summary of Benefits and Coverage (SBC) the ACA requires is your new best friend.

The SBC is a form that every insurance plan is required to use going forward so you can understand your current coverage and/or what you're considering buying. It's similar to the Nutrition Facts label you see on packaged foods. You can compare plans "apples to apples" because the information for each plan is laid out in the same way, using language that you can understand.

Each SBC gives you straightforward, easy-to-understand information about what your insurance covers, what it doesn't, and how much you pay. The federal government developed a template for the SBC that all insurers must use so you can make apples-to-apples comparisons among plans. The template requires that the insurer tell you these details:

- ✔ The plan's overall deductible
- ✔ Other deductibles that may apply for special services
- ✔ Any out-of-pocket limits on your expenses
- ✔ Items that aren't included in your out-of-pocket limit
- ✔ The annual limit on what the plan pays (if there is one)
- ✔ Whether the plan uses a network of providers
- ✔ Whether you must request a referral to see a specialist
- ✔ Any services that the plan doesn't cover

The SBC then lists common medical events (such as visiting a doctor's office, needing prescription drugs, and having outpatient surgery) and asks the insurer to tell you what your costs would be if you used an in-network provider and an out-of-network provider, as well as what limitations or exceptions may exist in the plan related to those events. There are also examples that show how the plan would cover two specific situations: a normal birth and management of type 2 diabetes. Since all plans have to use the same example, it may help consumers see how the coverage works.

Getting Signed Up

Before we walk through the *how* of enrolling in a Marketplace health plan, we want to explain the *when.* The Marketplace is always open for people who have certain major life events and need to change their coverage. In addition, each year eligible people have an open enrollment period during which they can make any changes to their coverage they'd like. In this section, we begin with when to sign up and then move on to the basics of getting signed up for a plan.

Understanding enrollment periods

Two types of enrollment periods exist:

- ✔ **Open enrollment:** This term refers to the time each year when anyone who needs coverage or wants to switch to a new insurance plan can enroll on the Marketplace. When the Marketplace first went live in fall 2013, that open enrollment period was set to last six months to accommodate the millions of people applying for coverage.

  As of 2014, the Marketplace allows open enrollment for a few months every year for signing up for coverage the following year. For example, for 2015 insurance coverage, open enrollment is slated to run from November 15, 2014, to January 15, 2015.

- ✔ **Special enrollment:** If you experience a *qualifying life event,* such as a job loss, a divorce, a marriage, the loss of your spouse, or the birth of a child, you have 60 days to shop for a new plan on the Marketplace, regardless of whether the event happens during an open enrollment period.

Getting Marketplace help

If you run into any trouble or have any uncertainty while you're creating a Marketplace account, filling out an application for coverage, shopping among your plan options, or enrolling, get customer service help these ways:

✔ Call 800-318-2596, 24 hours a day, 7 days a week. If you use a TTY, call 855-889-4325.

✔ Use the online chat function, which is also available 24/7. Locate the blue box in the lower-right corner of most Healthcare.gov pages, and type your question to have an online conversation with a Marketplace representative.

Keep in mind that if your state runs its own Marketplace, you'll be directed there for help.

If you prefer to speak to someone in your local area, go to LocalHelp.HealthCare.gov and type in your city and state or zip code. The site then pulls up a list of local organizations with contact information, office hours, and types of help offered. For example, you may find listings for entities that specialize in non-English language support, Medicaid or CHIP, and the Small Business Health Options Program (SHOP).

If you're already insured and are looking to change your coverage, you must wait until open enrollment. However, if your existing coverage changes during the year — for example, your employer decides to cut your hours and you no longer qualify for coverage — that event could qualify you for special enrollment if you choose to change plans.

If you have insurance through Medicare, that coverage is independent of the Health Insurance Marketplace. Medicare open enrollment occurs every year from October 15 to December 7.

Creating an account

Before you can start comparing the plans offered on your state's Marketplace, you must go through a simple process to create a Marketplace account. (Some states let you do a broad comparison of plans without setting up an account, but you won't get specific costs related to your characteristics, such as your age, family size, or tobacco use.) You provide basic information such as your name and contact information, and then you create a user name and password. You also select some security questions that help protect access to your account. Then you're ready to fill out an application for coverage.

Applying

You complete an application before you go shopping for plans. The information you provide in your applications helps the Marketplace determine which plans meet your needs.

The Marketplace application form has just three pages for individuals and seven pages for families, which is much shorter than the typical insurance form. To see the family application form, go to http://Marketplace.cms.gov/getofficialresources/publications-and-articles/Marketplace-application-for-family.pdf.

Print out the application first and review it in advance of applying. Before you apply, gather this information so you have an easier experience filling out the application:

- ✔ Social Security numbers for yourself and your family members

- ✔ Employer and income information for all members of your family (in the form of pay stubs, W-2 forms, or tax documents, for example)

- ✔ The policy number of your current insurance plan, if you have one

- ✔ Information about any employer-offered insurance you may be eligible to use

As we note earlier in the chapter, you can apply either online at healthcare.gov or, if you don't have computer access, by telephone (24 hours a day) at 800-318-2596. If you have a computer but prefer not to fill out the application online, you can print (or request by phone) a paper copy to fill out and return.

After you complete your application, you learn what financial help you qualify for. Be sure to provide all the information the application form requests so you can get the financial information you need without delay.

Appealing your eligibility

After you submit an application, you find out whether you qualify for financial support for purchasing an insurance plan (see Chapter 4). If the answer you get surprises you and doesn't seem right, you can file an appeal. Go to your Marketplace account at `HealthCare.gov/marketplace/individual` to start the process, or call the Marketplace at 800-318-2596 (or 855-889-4325 if you use a TTY). You can also mail an appeal form or your own letter filing an appeal to Health Insurance Marketplace, 465 Industrial Blvd., London, KY 40750-0061. You can ask a friend, relative, or lawyer to help with the appeal process, or you can do it yourself.

Selecting a plan

After you submit your application and you've had the opportunity to compare plans that are appropriate for you, you make your choice. Be certain that, before you do, you've found answers to all your questions about the new plan, such as "Can I still use my current doctor?" and "Will I be covered when I travel?" If the SBC for the plan doesn't spell out all the answers you need, ask for help from a Marketplace customer service representative, who can help you find what you need.

What happens if you choose your plan and go through the enrollment process, and then you decide you want to switch to another coverage option? It depends. If you change your mind immediately — before your coverage begins — and you're still within an enrollment period (either open or special enrollment), you should be able to make the change by revisiting the Marketplace. However, if your coverage has already started when you change your mind, you must wait until the next open enrollment period to make a change (unless you experience a qualifying event before that, in which case you can change during a special enrollment period).

Enrolling

You enroll by selecting the plan you want to purchase and making arrangements to pay for it. This step is fairly quick and easy.

If you qualify for tax credits that help offset your premium costs (see Chapter 4), after you enroll, you can have those credits sent directly to the insurance company to reduce the premium you owe. You then arrange to pay the premium in a way that's the most convenient to you, whether online or by mail.

Note that you make your premium payments to the insurance company itself, not to the Marketplace in your state. After you enroll, you're directed to the insurer's own website to make your first payment. Under the ACA, insurers must work with various forms of payment (including paper checks and money orders); you cannot be forced to have a credit card or bank account.

You need to send in your first payment so it's processed at least a day before your coverage is set to start. Before you enroll, you'll know the premium due dates for that plan so you can anticipate when your first and subsequent payments are needed. If you cannot locate this information or you have any doubts about it, be sure to ask a Marketplace customer service representative for assistance.

After you've paid your first month's premium, if you're getting tax credits to help pay for your coverage, your insurer must grant you a 90-day grace period if you're late with a subsequent premium payment. You must get current with your premium payments within those 90 days to avoid having your coverage canceled. Thirty days into that grace period, the insurer has the right to withhold payment for any new claims. That means if your policy is terminated because you don't pay your premiums in full, you're on the hook for services you used in the final two months of the grace period. (The grace period for people who don't receive tax credit assistance is generally much shorter.)

The bottom line is this: Before you enroll, make sure you're committed to making your premium payments on time. Otherwise, you may be digging yourself a financial hole and jeopardizing your ability to maintain coverage and comply with the ACA.

Chapter 3

Knowing What You're Buying

. . . .

In This Chapter

▶ Getting familiar with coverage and benefits

▶ Identifying types of insurance plans available

▶ Understanding the metal categories: bronze, silver, gold, and platinum

▶ Steering clear of scams

. . . .

*T*his chapter is a must-read, whether or not you already
have insurance. We start with an overview of some of the
most important information every American needs to know
about how the Affordable Care Act affects private health
insurance coverage. Because of the ACA, many private insurance policies (meaning those not run by the government)
must provide certain essential benefits, and we explain them
here so you know what to expect from your coverage going
forward.

If you aren't insured and you need to go shopping for a policy
on the Health Insurance Marketplace (which we introduce
in Chapter 2), the rest of this chapter walks you through the
types of plan options available there. You find out how an
HMO differs from a PPO, as well as what it means to buy a
bronze, silver, gold, or platinum plan.

Finally, you get some advice for avoiding scams while you're
shopping for coverage. Unfortunately, any significant change
in federal law brings out the worst in a small number of people
who want to play on fear and uncertainty for their own profit.
Don't lose one dime to a scam artist: Read the advice in this
chapter, and be informed and alert.

Identifying the Essential Health Benefits Covered

Under the ACA, all new health plans sold to individuals and small groups, whether through the Health Insurance Marketplace or not, must provide certain types of coverage that are detailed in this section.

To be clear, all nongrandfathered individual and *small group market* plans — employer-provided insurance plans offered by companies with 50 or fewer full-time equivalent employees — must offer this coverage as of 2014. (A *nongrandfathered* plan is not exempt from any of the ACA's provisions. For more on grandfathered plans, see Chapter 1.) All grandfathered large group, small group, and individual plans are currently exempt from this ACA provision. But because grandfathered plans can make only very limited changes to the benefits and premiums they had in place in 2010 or lose their grandfathered status, it's anticipated that there will be increasingly fewer grandfathered plans.

If you shop for a plan on the Marketplace, or if you work for a small business that offers coverage through the SHOP Marketplace (see Chapter 6), this section contains helpful information about what your insurance coverage must offer. (New individual and small group plans purchased via insurance agents and brokers must offer the same.) Of course, your plan may offer *more* than these essential benefits, so don't consider this information a substitute for your specific plan's details.

Preventive and wellness care

Many people have important preventive and wellness benefits because of the ACA — with no deductibles and copayments.

The ACA provides for an annual well-woman visit for adult women under age 65 so that they and their doctors can determine what preventive services may be needed.

All plans offered in the Marketplace, as well as any individual and small group insurance plans that aren't grandfathered per the ACA, must also provide important preventive services at no additional cost to you — even if your plan has a deductible that you haven't yet met. Although the ACA encourages prevention by removing your costs for some services, it isn't a perfect solution. You may be responsible for costs related to a service — for example, a facility or office fee — even if there is no cost for you for the screening test itself. And if the screening results in diagnostic services – for example, the doctor finds polyps during a routine colonoscopy – you may be charged for their removal and biopsy.

To tap into these preventive services without paying anything out of pocket, you likely need to use an in-network health provider. Be sure to read the details of your own insurance policy to determine how to identify in-network providers in your area.

Preventive screenings the ACA covers may change over time, but they now include the following:

- Blood pressure, for every adult

- Cholesterol, for older adults or people at higher risk

- Colorectal cancer, for people over age 50

- Depression, for every adult

- Diabetes Type 2, for any adult with high blood pressure

- HIV, for anyone age 15 to 65 (and at other ages for people who have evidence of increased risk)

For women, additional preventive screenings are covered, including the following:

- Anemia, gestational diabetes, Rh incompatibility, and hepatitis B, for women who are pregnant

- Cervical cancer, for women who are sexually active

- Mammography, for every woman over age 40

- Osteoporosis, for women over age 60 who are at risk

Other screenings are available to women at risk for sexually transmitted diseases; counseling is offered to women with a higher risk of developing breast cancer; and some forms of contraception, including education and counseling, are offered to all women who could become pregnant. Verify what is covered by your plan and any associated costs.

In addition, the ACA covers screening and counseling for men and women who use alcohol or tobacco products, diet counseling for adults who are at higher risk for developing chronic illness, and obesity screening and counseling for all adults.

Many immunization vaccines are also available with no costs to you. The ACA covers vaccines for flu; measles, mumps, and rubella; hepatitis A and B; pneumonia; and more.

As Chapter 2 details, the ACA requires your insurer to give you a Summary of Benefits and Coverage (SBC) — a document that spells out your benefits and coverage in language that's easy to understand. If you're shopping for coverage and want to know what a certain plan covers, or if you already have insurance and want to know which preventive services you can expect, check the SBC.

Pediatric care

Under the ACA, many health plans — including Medicaid and all insurance plans sold through the Marketplace — must cover certain preventive services for children at no cost to you (even if you haven't yet met your plan's deductible). Again, check your plan's SBC for your specific coverage, but here are some of the essentials the ACA provides for:

- ✔ Autism screening at 18 and 24 months
- ✔ Behavioral assessments at various recommended ages
- ✔ Blood pressure screenings at various recommended ages
- ✔ Depression screening for adolescents
- ✔ Developmental screenings for children under age 3
- ✔ Hearing and sickle cell screenings for all newborns
- ✔ Height, weight, and body mass measurements
- ✔ Hematocrit or hemoglobin screening
- ✔ Oral health risk assessment at various recommended ages
- ✔ Vision screenings for all children

In addition, children with specific risks are entitled to the following benefits:

- ✔ Fluoride supplements
- ✔ Iron supplements
- ✔ Obesity screening and counseling
- ✔ Screening for lead exposure
- ✔ Screening for lipid disorders
- ✔ Tuberculosis testing

The ACA also provides that children receive recommended vaccinations at no cost to you, including for flu; measles, mumps, and rubella; rotavirus; hepatitis A and B; diphtheria, tetanus, and pertussis; and human papillomavirus (HPV).

Prescription drugs

Before the passage of the ACA, many insurance plans offered prescription drug coverage only as an option at extra cost to you. But because of the ACA, all nongrandfathered individual and small-group plans, including all of those offered on the Marketplace, must provide prescription coverage.

The ACA specifically states that insurers must cover at least one drug in every category and class listed in the *U.S. Pharmacopeia,* which is an official publication of approved medications in the United States. This means that you may not get insurance coverage for a brand-name drug if your coverage instead applies to its generic equivalent. Your insurer can give you a list (called a *formulary*) of the drugs your plan covers. When in doubt, speak with your doctor and/or pharmacist before you have a prescription ordered so you can take full advantage of this benefit.

Keep in mind that this benefit doesn't mean that your prescription drugs will be free. Instead, your health plan must offer coverage that amounts to a discounted out-of-pocket price for you. Per the ACA, any money you pay out of pocket for prescription drugs must count toward your out-of-pocket caps on medical expenses.

The ACA deals with contraceptives slightly differently than other prescription drugs. Unless you have coverage through a grandfathered plan or you work for a religious entity that opposes birth control use, your insurance should provide some contraceptive options at no cost to you. Not every contraceptive may be covered, however. If a generic option of the birth control pill is covered at no cost to you, for example, a brand-name option may involve out-of-pocket expenses. If you have any questions about what your plan does and doesn't provide for, check with your plan.

Lab services

As outlined in the "Preventive and wellness care" section earlier in the chapter, the ACA spells out which preventive screening tests must be covered by nongrandfathered individual and small-group plans, including all those sold on the Marketplace. You aren't required to pay any out-of-pocket costs for these essential screenings.

However, when you have symptoms of disease, or if you're seeking information about potential risks for disease, your doctor may order diagnostic tests that aren't included in the list of fully covered screenings per the ACA. In this case, your plan needs to spell out your coverage, which may require a copayment (a flat rate cost) or coinsurance (a percentage cost) that you must pay out of pocket. For example, if your doctor orders a CAT scan of your liver, your plan may require you to pay 30 percent of its total cost. Or if your doctor orders blood work that isn't covered by the preventive screenings, you may have a flat copay, such as $20, for that test.

 Keep in mind that many lab services involve out-of-pocket expenses, even though the ACA requires plans to offer lab coverage. Have your insurance plan's SBC handy to help you anticipate laboratory costs.

Emergency services

Even before the ACA, most health insurance plans provided some form of coverage for visits to a hospital emergency room. So what's different under the ACA? The law has two key provisions that improve emergency care:

✔ **Emergency room visits don't require preauthorization.** Insurers can't require that you contact them before using emergency services. So if you or your spouse is experiencing signs of a stroke, for example, and you call an ambulance, you don't have to fear that your insurer will later refuse to pay any associated bills because you didn't call to ask for permission to seek care.

✔ **Your insurer must provide the same copayment amount or coinsurance percentage, regardless of which emergency health provider you use, in or out of network.** This provision is especially important for anyone who travels. If you're away from home and experience an emergency, you cannot be penalized for seeking care out of town or out of state, regardless of which emergency health provider you use.

As with the other provisions outlined in this section, this one applies to individual and small-group plans that aren't grandfathered, including all those sold on the Marketplace. Check your plan's SBC to find out what you can expect to pay for emergency care.

Ambulatory patient services

Don't let the term confuse you: *Ambulatory* doesn't involve an ambulance. This phrase refers to outpatient care — the kind you get whenever you walk into a doctor's office or an urgent care facility, get treated for some kind of ailment, and walk back out. The ACA doesn't have a tremendous impact on outpatient services because almost all health insurance plans already provided this type of coverage before its passage.

To pay the least out-of-pocket expenses for outpatient care, you generally need to visit a doctor who's in your plan's network. Be sure to check your plan details (starting with its SBC) to find out how to locate an in-network provider. For more information about networks and how they impact your coverage, check out the upcoming section "Alphabet Soup: Selecting the Type of Plan You Need."

Hospitalization

As with outpatient care, most insurance policies offered coverage for the costs of hospitalization even before the ACA. The ACA does stipulate that insurers must provide minimum essential coverage, however, which means that certain types of hospitalization policies aren't sufficient.

For example, a plan that limits coverage to a set dollar amount each day (an *indemnity* plan) isn't considered sufficient coverage by itself, per the ACA. You may want to purchase an indemnity plan to supplement your existing insurance, but that type of plan alone doesn't provide the minimum essential coverage the law requires.

Another example is insurance that covers hospital expenses only for a certain disease, such as cancer. On its own, that type of policy isn't considered sufficient coverage because it won't help you if you're hospitalized for any other reason.

Your insurance policy isn't required to pay 100 percent of your expenses related to a hospitalization, and it likely won't pay that much. If you haven't reached your out-of-pocket expense limit for the year, you can expect to pay a share of the bill. It may be a big chunk of change if you're hospitalized for a long period of time. Don't be caught by surprise: Read your policy carefully, starting with the SBC, to find out what to expect if you're hospitalized.

Maternity and newborn care

Before the ACA, many people got a nasty surprise when they discovered that their insurance policies excluded prenatal and maternity care. (As many as two-thirds of plans did so.) Under the ACA, prenatal care is classified as a preventive service that must be provided at no extra cost as part of nongrandfathered individual and small-group plans. As we note in the "Preventive and wellness care" section earlier in the chapter, this fact means that a pregnant woman receives standard screenings, such as screenings for anemia, gestational diabetes, Rh incompatibility, and hepatitis B, at no cost to her.

In addition, the ACA requires that health plans cover expenses related to childbirth, as well as the newborn infant's care. Keep in mind that insurers aren't required to offer 100 percent coverage for childbirth expenses, so you can expect some out-of-pocket costs, depending on your specific plan. But plans must cover newborn screenings and tests that are considered essential preventive care at no additional expense to the parents; refer to the "Preventive and wellness care" section.

If you have health insurance and are looking to change plans, keep in mind that you can go shopping for new coverage after the birth of a child, or you can add the child to your existing coverage. That event qualifies as a special enrollment opportunity, which means you have 60 days to purchase new coverage. However, pregnancy itself doesn't qualify as a special enrollment opportunity; you can't go shopping for new coverage after you get pregnant (unless you experience some other event, such as a job loss or loss of a spouse, that triggers a special enrollment opportunity). See Chapter 2 for a discussion of enrollment periods.

Mental health care

Before the ACA was signed into law, many health insurance plans didn't cover mental or behavioral health services at all. Now, such services are considered to be essential health benefits that any nongrandfathered individual or small-group plan (including all plans sold on the Marketplace) must offer. Such services aren't required to be covered at 100 percent, so you may pay out-of-pocket expenses, such as copayments for office visits, just as with the medical care you receive.

Keep in mind that mental health care receives the same protections as other healthcare (see Chapter 1).

- ✔ Insurers must cover preexisting mental health conditions.

- ✔ An insurer cannot cancel your coverage if you develop a mental health issue that requires services.

- ✔ Insurers cannot impose annual or lifetime limits on mental health coverage (meaning that your policy can't be canceled after you use a certain threshold of services).

- ✔ An insurer must offer mental health service benefits that are on par with other medical service benefits. In other words, if your insurance plan doesn't limit how many medical doctor visits it covers in a given year, it cannot limit how many visits to a mental health provider it covers. If it does establish limits on medical care, it can create similar limits with mental health care.

Rehabilitative and habilitative services

To understand what insurers must cover, first let's define these terms:

- ✔ **Rehabilitative:** These services help a patient who has been sick, hurt, or disabled to retain or regain skills or functions that are required for everyday life. Such services help relieve pain and support the ability to speak and walk, for example; they include coverage for canes, walkers, wheelchairs, and other devices that improve mobility.

- ✔ **Habilitative:** These services are therapies that aim to help someone overcome a long-term disability. For example, someone who has Parkinson's disease or multiple sclerosis may use habilitative services to try to retain the skills and functions he currently has and possibly try to regain some he has lost. A child with developmental delays that affect her skill development may also use habilitative services.

In the past, health insurance plans often offered coverage for rehabilitative services but rarely did for habilitative services. Today, all Marketplace and nongrandfathered individual and small-group insurance policies must cover both. Check the SBC for your policy (or the policy you're considering buying) to find out what that coverage looks like and what to expect for out-of-pocket costs.

Dental and vision care for children

The earlier section "Pediatric care" outlines the essential medical benefits for children that the ACA requires. In addition, children under age 19 now have greater access to basic dental and vision services. All nongrandfathered individual and small-group plans must provide these services either within the plan itself or via an add-on plan.

Through this coverage, children can generally get their teeth cleaned twice a year and receive X-rays, fillings, and medically necessary orthodontia. Children under age 19 are also entitled to one eye exam and one pair of glasses or set of contact lenses each year.

If you have an existing individual or small-group plan and haven't heard about these benefits available to your children, ask for the plan's SBC and find out whether your plan is providing this coverage itself or is offering you a separate policy to meet this coverage.

Alphabet Soup: Selecting the Type of Plan You Need

If you've ever had to choose between two or more insurance plan options at work, or if you've ever gone shopping for health coverage as an individual, you know that deciphering insurance-speak isn't always easy. The ACA helps consumers by pushing insurers toward greater clarity, requiring that they use a template to present easy-to-read information in the SBC. But the healthcare jargon doesn't entirely go away.

This section quickly runs through the basics to keep in mind regarding the broad types of private insurance plans available (both through employers and on the Marketplace). With this information squared away in your mind, you'll be a more informed consumer whether you're shopping for new health coverage or simply trying to decipher what you already have.

HMOs and EPOs

A *health maintenance organization* (HMO) and an *exclusive provider organization* (EPO) have a lot in common. Both types of insurance plans require that you seek healthcare within a network of providers if you want to tap into the plan's coverage. A *network* refers to the healthcare providers, such as doctors, laboratories, and hospitals, that have agreed to provide their services to people with your insurance plan.

What happens if you go outside the network to get care? You'll pay more out-of-pocket costs, possibly even the entire amount. For this reason, when you're shopping for an HMO or EPO, you absolutely need to know whether the network providers include the doctors, lab, and hospital you're most likely to use.

The key difference between these two types of network plans is that HMOs usually require that you get a referral if you need to see a specialist, whereas EPOs generally don't.

PPOs and POS plans

With a *preferred provider organization* (PPO) or a *point-of-service* (POS) plan, your coverage isn't restricted to a network of service providers. You have more freedom to choose your doctors, hospital, and so on than you have with an HMO or EPO. However, you're still rewarded for staying within the network because your out-of-pocket costs will be higher if you go outside the network for care.

With a PPO, you're able to get coverage for any doctor you see, even if you don't have a referral. A POS allows you to see any in-network doctor without a referral, but if you want to go outside the network, you need a referral if you want the plan to cover the visit. Plans vary, so check with your plan before you use an out-of-network provider.

HDHPs

A *high deductible health plan* (HDHP) has a lower premium than traditional insurance. It also has a higher deductible. For example, for a family plan, an HDHP may have a $2,500 deductible, which means that if you seek any service other than the preventive care services that are wholly covered under the ACA, you'll pay a lot of costs before your plan benefits kick in.

People using these plans may have a health savings account (HSA) or health reimbursement arrangement (HRA), to help them pay for health expenses. When you incur a qualified healthcare expense, you can pay for it (or be reimbursed) from that account. An HSA may decrease your federal tax burden for the year.

Catastrophic plans

A catastrophic plan can be purchased only by someone who is under age 30 or someone who can't find a plan in the Marketplace that costs less than 8 percent of his or her income or who can't afford more coverage because of a hardship.

Catastrophic plans can be purchased both in the Marketplace and outside of it (through an insurance agent or broker).

These plans must cover the essential health benefits outlined at the beginning of this chapter, but they feature a very high deductible (in the thousands of dollars for an individual) that applies to benefits other than preventive and wellness care and three primary care visits a year. So although the coverage provided may not differ greatly from another plan offered on the Marketplace, the amount you pay before coverage actually kicks in may be significantly different.

In 2014, the annual deductible for covered services under this type of policy is $6,350 for an individual and $12,700 for a family. After you satisfy the deductible, the plan pays 100 percent for covered essential health benefit services for the rest of the year.

As the name implies, this type of plan is essentially the bare-bones coverage you can get to support you in case catastrophe strikes (you have a bad accident or you're diagnosed with a serious chronic illness, for example). It qualifies as sufficient coverage per the ACA because the elements of coverage are intact; you just may not ever tap into some of them because your out-of-pocket costs would need to be very high to do so.

In Chapter 4, we explain that many people are eligible (based on their household incomes) for discounted, or subsidized, premiums and/or out-of-pocket costs if they purchase coverage through the Marketplace. However, *someone who purchases a catastrophic plan isn't eligible for those subsidies*; only someone purchasing a metal plan, which we explain next, can qualify for financial assistance.

Going for a Bronze, Silver, Gold, or Platinum Plan

If you shop on the Health Insurance Marketplace, which Chapter 2 outlines, you'll find that the plans available to you are labeled by type of metal: bronze, silver, gold, or platinum. (If you're under age 30 or you're unable to find coverage in the Marketplace that costs less than 8 percent of your income, you can also consider catastrophic plans, which we explain in the previous section.)

The metals represent various levels of coverage you receive and what the plan pays on average. The plan levels do *not* represent the quality of the health coverage you receive. As we explain earlier in this chapter, the ACA requires that all Marketplace plans offer essential health benefits, including preventive and wellness care, at no additional charge to you. While Marketplace plans certainly may differ from each other in the types of additional coverage offered, the metal designations are used strictly to highlight how you and the insurance company share costs for a plan — not to indicate the plan's quality.

Here's the rundown:

- **Bronze:** If you buy into a bronze plan, you can expect to pay, in general, relatively low premiums, but out-of-pocket costs, in the form of copayments, coinsurance, and deductibles, are the highest among all four categories. Bronze plans cover approximately 60 percent of healthcare costs, and individuals are responsible for approximately 40 percent. Therefore, a bronze plan likely makes most sense for someone who isn't expecting to use health services often during the year.

- **Silver:** A silver plan's premium generally is higher than that of a bronze plan, and its out-of-pocket costs are lower. Silver plans cover approximately 70 percent of healthcare costs, and individuals are responsible for approximately 30 percent.

- **Gold:** A gold plan's premium generally is higher than that of a silver plan, and its out-of-pocket costs are lower. Gold plans cover approximately 80 percent of healthcare costs, and individuals are responsible for approximately 20 percent.

- **Platinum:** A platinum plan's premiums generally are the highest among the metal levels, and its out-of-pocket costs are lowest. Platinum plans cover approximately 90 percent of healthcare costs, and individuals are responsible for approximately 10 percent. Whereas a bronze plan may make sense for a healthy person who anticipates needing little medical care, a platinum plan may make good sense for someone who expects to need ongoing and/or intensive health services.

How significant are the differences in premiums among the various metal plans? You can answer that question only by checking out your state's Marketplace offerings; visit www.healthcare.gov/what-is-the-marketplace-in-my-state to get started. Broadly speaking, you can pay up to a few thousand dollars more annually for premiums for a platinum plan than for a bronze plan. Is it worth the upfront expense to do so? That answer depends entirely on your healthcare needs and the out-of-pocket costs you may face if selecting a bronze plan.

The U.S. government has established financial subsidies to help individuals who purchase insurance via the online Marketplace. If your income qualifies for this assistance, you must enroll in a metal plan (not a catastrophic plan) to get a tax credit to help pay your insurance premiums. If you qualify to reduce your out-of-pocket expenses as well, you must enroll specifically in a silver (midlevel) plan. We explain both types of potential cost savings in Chapter 4.

Being on the Lookout for Scams

Since the ACA was passed in 2010, periodic waves of cons tied to health reform have reared their ugly heads. These include the sale of bogus insurance policies, as well as phone calls demanding sensitive personal information if you're to receive a (nonexistent) Obamacare card or a new Medicare card.

Confusion over the ACA certainly helps the con artists, so you're taking a great step by reading this book. Many people are unaware of what they need to do (or don't need to do) to comply with the ACA.

Some scammers have established fake websites claiming to sell ACA insurance. Others have renewed tried-and-true government impostor scams — delivered via phone call, fax, and e-mail — in which they claim to represent Medicare or other government agencies, sometimes just saying they're "calling from Obamacare." The goal is to get sensitive information for identity theft while pitching phony health plan enrollments.

Here are key pieces of information to help you keep scammers at bay:

✔ If you have Medicare, you don't need a new card or additional insurance because of the ACA. (See Chapter 5 for an overview of how the ACA and Medicare interact.)

✔ As always, you can change your Medicare plan and prescription coverage during Medicare open enrollment from mid-October through early December each year, but no one from Medicare — or any other federal office — will make unsolicited contact via telephone, e-mail, fax, or a front-door visit. If anyone reaches out to you to ask for money or personal or financial information, including your Social Security/Medicare number, that person does *not* work for the U.S. government.

✔ If you get health insurance at work, your employer should notify you — via official workplace correspondence — of what, if any, changes may occur. If you have private insurance through your employer, contact your human resources department; if you buy insurance on your own, contact your insurance provider with any questions.

✔ You don't need to pay anyone a single cent to help you sign up for health benefits, whether you're applying for a public (government) program for the first time or shopping for private coverage.

✔ Most people who need insurance are shopping on the federal or state Health Insurance Marketplace websites (see Chapter 2), but legitimate insurance vendors may reach out to you via phone or e-mail. (No one is required to purchase insurance via the Marketplace; you can still get a policy through an insurance agent or broker, or directly from an insurance company.)

If someone calls you offering to sell you insurance, ask to receive information in the mail before you try to determine whether it's a legitimate offer. If you receive an e-mail offering coverage, don't click on any links included in the e-mail. Check first to make sure the vendor is legitimate and that the vendor actually sent the e-mail.

To help answer questions about plans you may consider, as well as vendor and product legitimacy, you can contact the federal government's hotline, 800-318-2596 (TTY 855-889-3425), or visit healthcare.gov. Do so before you provide sensitive details or sign anything.

✔ A Health Insurance Marketplace website for any state ends in ".gov," as does the federal website, healthcare.gov. If you receive communication suggesting that you visit a Marketplace website with an address that doesn't end in ".gov," stay away so you don't accidentally download any malware onto your computer.

✔ Although some states have enlisted advertisers and translators to help educate residents about new benefits for the uninsured, their role is strictly to educate consumers — not to sell policies.

✔ Scare or rush tactics signal you're dealing with a scammer. Claims of "limited-time offers" and "act now or lose benefits" are lies.

✔ Scammers like to go after your medical records, called "fulls" in scammer jargon because they provide everything in one place for ID theft. Fetching as much as 50 times the rate of a Social Security number on online black markets, a stolen medical record opens the way for scammers to pose as you and to buy medications or to pay for medical treatments. And unlike in the case of credit card theft, victims may be responsible for these charges and may lose their coverage. So guard details of your medical history, treatments, or insurance — no matter what you're being offered in return.

If you believe you've been contacted by a scammer, law enforcement officials need you to report your concerns. The ACA includes extra resources for fighting healthcare fraud. Contact your state insurance commission, your state attorney general, or local law enforcement about any suspicious promotions. You can find contact information for your state insurance commission at www.naic.org/state_web_map.htm. You can locate your state attorney general at www.naag.org/current-attorneys-general.php. Report Medicare fraud to Medicare at 800-MEDICARE (800-633-4227). You can find more information about healthcare fraud and scams at www.aarp.org/fightfraud.

Chapter 4

Controlling Your Costs

. . . .

In This Chapter

▶ Securing and maintaining coverage

▶ Estimating your out-of-pocket costs

▶ Getting financial assistance through a tax credit

▶ Seeking help for out-of-pocket costs

▶ Keeping taxes in check if your income is higher

. . . .

*T*he ACA aims to get more people covered so they can get access to health care and improve the quality of health-care people receive.

In this chapter, we consolidate information about the financial aspects of complying with the ACA: how to secure and maintain coverage, what you can expect if you don't purchase insurance, how to get a sense of the costs and options as you select a plan a plan, the types of financial assistance you may qualify to receive from the federal government depending on your income, and what steps you may want to take if your income is fairly high to anticipate or avoid tax consequences.

Understanding the Consequences of Not Carrying Coverage

Under the ACA, every American is required to have what's called *minimum essential coverage* through a healthcare plan. That coverage can take many forms, including the following:

  ✔ An employer-sponsored plan, including COBRA and retiree coverage.

- ✔ An individual plan purchased in the Health Insurance Marketplace (also called the *exchange*).

- ✔ Medicare, Medicaid, or CHIP (Children's Health Insurance Program) coverage.

- ✔ TRICARE, which covers uniformed military personnel.

- ✔ Some plans administered by the Veterans Administration.

- ✔ Coverage for Peace Corps volunteers.

- ✔ Self-funded health coverage plans that universities offer to students for plan or policy years that begin on or before December 31, 2014. (Starting in 2015, these types of plans may or may not count as minimum essential coverage; they must demonstrate to the federal government that they are sufficient.)

- ✔ State high-risk pools for plan or policy years that begin on or before December 31, 2014. (Starting in 2015, these types of plans also may or may not count as minimum essential coverage.)

If you have existing coverage that falls into one of these categories, you're likely good to go. If you don't, keep in mind that insurance plans that provide only limited benefits, such as vision or dental care, don't qualify as minimum essential coverage, nor do workers' compensation or disability policies. Even some Medicaid coverage, if it applies only to specific benefits such as family planning or pregnancy-related services, doesn't suffice.

Qualifying for an exemption

In Chapter 1, we explain that certain groups of people are exempt from the requirement that all individuals secure health coverage. Here are the exempt groups as of this writing:

- ✔ People who are incarcerated

- ✔ Members of federally recognized Indian tribes

- ✔ People who are part of a healthcare sharing ministry or a recognized religious sect with objections to health insurance

> ✔ Non–U.S. citizens, U.S. nationals, and resident aliens law-fully present in the United States
>
> ✔ People who cannot qualify for Medicaid because their state has chosen not to expand the program (see Chapter 1)
>
> ✔ Anyone who cannot afford coverage, which means they would pay more than 8 percent of their household income for the lowest-cost bronze plan available to them through the Marketplace
>
> ✔ People whose income is low enough that they aren't required to file a federal tax return

You can file for an exemption on your state's Health Insurance Marketplace or when you file your federal tax return. If you aren't required to file a federal return, you are automatically exempt from the insurance mandate that year.

Facing the consequences

If you aren't exempt and you choose not to secure insurance coverage, you face tax penalties starting in 2014. In addition, you will have to pay all your health care costs and risk accruing debt and not receiving good health care. Medical expenses prompt most personal bankruptcies in the United States.

You may be assessed a tax penalty if you go without coverage for three or more consecutive months during the year. You're allowed to have one gap in coverage that lasts up to three months. If you have more than one such gap during the year, you're penalized for the subsequent gaps.

Keep in mind that this provision also applies to children. If you're a parent or can otherwise claim someone as a dependent on your federal income tax return, you owe the tax penalty for your dependent who doesn't have insurance coverage (or isn't part of an exempt group).

You are charged the higher of these two amounts:

> ✔ **A percentage of your annual household income:** This fee is determined based on the number of months during the year that you go without coverage (or without an exemption). You pay the fee when you pay your federal income tax.

In 2014, this fee equals 1 percent of your household income (minus the federal tax filing threshold, which, in 2014, is $10,000 for an individual or $20,000 for a couple filing jointly). The percentage is set to increase each year so it becomes a bigger deterrent to ignoring the law. In 2015, it equates to 2 percent of your household income, and in 2016, it increases to 2.5 percent.

✔ **A flat rate:** This rate is also assessed on a monthly basis and is set to increase each year. In 2014, the flat rate equals $95 per person, per year, and $47.50 per child under 18 per year. Per family, the 2014 cap is $285 per year. You pay according to the number of months you lack coverage or an exemption during the year. (You're allowed one gap of up to three months before you need to pay the penalty.)

The flat rate jumps substantially after 2014. For example, in 2015, the family penalty is $975; in 2016, it's $2,085. Again, the idea is to increase tax penalties over time to encourage the greatest possible participation in sharing healthcare costs.

Regardless of which amount is higher, your tax penalty is capped at a dollar figure equivalent to that year's national average annual premium for the lowest-cost bronze plan on the Health Insurance Marketplace. (We explain plan levels in Chapter 3.)

But you want to keep something else in mind: Even if you pay a tax penalty for not securing coverage (or an exemption), you are still on the hook for medical expenses you incur while you lack coverage. Your tax penalty doesn't constitute insurance coverage.

Obviously, if you don't currently have the minimum essential insurance coverage the ACA requires, your best bet is to get obtain coverage. If you qualify for an exemption, apply for it (unless your income is low enough that you don't file federal income taxes). If you aren't exempt, go on the Marketplace and get coverage. If the cost of buying insurance is too high, keep reading to find out what help is available — and keep the costs of *not* buying insurance clearly in sight.

Using Online Tools to Estimate Your Out-of-Pocket Costs

To know the exact amounts you'll pay for plans that fit your needs, you must apply to the Health Insurance Marketplace; we provide information in Chapter 2 on how to do so. But before you apply, you may be able to get a general sense of insurance plans offered in your area and how much they cost so you can begin to estimate what to expect.

The federal government's health insurance website is a place to start. Go to www.healthcare.gov/find-premium-estimates — you're asked to answer a few general questions about what you're looking for. Depending on the state where you live, you're either directed to the homepage for your state's Marketplace or you can view premium estimates based solely on your answers to the initial questions.

Keep in mind that the estimates reflect only monthly premiums — not any other out-of-pocket costs, such as deductibles, copayments, coinsurance, or out-of-network amounts. Information on other out-of-pocket costs is available at www.healthcare.gov.

Also keep in mind that the premiums you see at this step don't reflect your specific situation, including your annual household income. These premiums don't reflect any cost savings that may be available to many people based on income. Therefore, your actual cost may end up being much lower than what the estimate tools reflect. If your income level qualifies you for a financial subsidy in the form of tax credits (which we discuss in the next section), you may see substantial savings compared with the initial estimates.

Alternately, the estimates you view may be lower than your actual rates because you haven't added your specific personal information, such as your tobacco usage.

This tool is designed just to provide some examples of plans and premiums available in your area. When you actually apply to the Marketplace, the plans and premium prices shown to you will be tailored to the number of people in your household and their ages, your income, and whether any household members use tobacco.

So here's the million-dollar question (or at least the several-hundred-dollar question): Without applying to the Marketplace, how you can get a sense of whether your situation qualifies you for financial assistance? The Kaiser Family Foundation has created an online subsidy calculator that you can access at http://kff.org/interactive/subsidy-calculator/.

Much like the premium estimates tool, this subsidy calculator provides just a rough estimate. You don't know until you apply to the Marketplace exactly how much (if any) assistance you qualify for. Plus, the calculator bases its estimates on health insurance plans in the silver category (see Chapter 3), so your savings may differ significantly if you choose a plan from another category. But the calculator does account for some of the key factors that influence the cost of insurance plans on the Marketplace, such as the size of your household, your age, where you live, and whether anyone in your family uses tobacco.

Tapping into a Tax Credit

The ACA provides a tax credit, based on income, that helps lower premium costs for people who qualify. In this section, we explain how the credit works and how you determine whether you qualify for this financial assistance.

This tax credit is available to help people who the ACA requires to get coverage. If you have coverage that meets the ACA's standards for existing health coverage — whether through a government program such as Medicare, an employer-sponsored plan, or any other program — you don't have access to a tax credit.

Seeing how the credit works

When you submit a completed application to the Health Insurance Marketplace (a process we explain in Chapter 2), you find out whether your situation qualifies you for receiving reductions on monthly plan premiums. Premium tax credits are available to people whose modified adjusted gross income is between 100 percent and 400 percent of the federal poverty level. Both income and the cost of the insurance plans available on the Marketplace in your area determine the size of the tax credit. As you shop for plans (another subject we cover in Chapter 2), you'll see the lower costs reflected in the prices you're comparing.

The tax credit calculation works like this:

1. **Based on your income, the Marketplace figures out how much you'd be expected to contribute to the premiums for a silver insurance plan in your area.** In Chapter 3, we explain that you can choose among bronze, silver, gold, and platinum insurance plans. The silver is a midlevel plan: It doesn't have the highest premiums or the highest out-of-pocket costs.

   The calculation uses a sliding scale. If your income level equals 100 percent of the federal poverty level, you'd pay 2 percent of your income toward premiums. If you earn close to 400 percent of the federal poverty level, the expected contribution jumps to 9.5 percent of your income.

2. **The tax credit amount equals the difference between your expected contribution and the premium cost for the silver plan being used as a benchmark.** For example, if your expected contribution is $95 per month and the silver plan premium is $325 per month, your monthly tax credit is $230.

Even though your tax credit is calculated using a silver plan as a benchmark, you can apply the credit whether you purchase a bronze, silver, gold, or platinum plan. You cannot, however, use the tax credit if you purchase a catastrophic plan (see Chapter 3).

You have two ways to apply your tax credit:

✔ **Advanced premium tax credit:** You can have the credit applied directly to your plan premiums when you enroll. If you take this route, you don't need to wait until April 15 of the following year to see the benefits; your premium costs are lowered from the moment you sign up for a plan.

   If you choose this option, each month the federal government will send the monthly tax credit amount directly to your insurance company. The insurance company will then bill you for the remaining premium amount.

✔ **Premium tax credit:** Instead of receiving the entire tax credit in advance (applied to your premiums), you can wait until the end of the tax year to claim all or part of it. For example, you can choose to apply only a portion of the tax credit to your monthly premium and to take the rest of it as a credit when you file your federal tax return.

You may want to take this route if you aren't certain what your income will be in the following year. An advanced premium tax credit calculation is based on your estimated income for the year in which you need insurance coverage. If your income increases during the year and you've taken a higher tax credit than you're actually eligible for, you may need to pay back the excess you've used. You do this when you file your federal return, as well.

If you have a tax credit on the Marketplace and your income changes significantly during the year, you need to report the changes to the Marketplace. Otherwise, you'll be reporting the change after the fact and may need to repay tax credits.

The tax credit applies _only_ when you purchase a plan through the Marketplace. The ACA doesn't require that you purchase insurance through the Marketplace, but if you purchase an individual plan through an insurance company or broker, you cannot tap into cost savings through the tax credit.

Modified adjusted gross income

Figuring out your _modified adjusted gross income_ (MAGI) is necessary for determining tax credits. To calculate your MAGI, you first calculate your adjusted gross income. You add up your wages, salary, and tips; taxable interest; the taxable portion of a pension, annuity, IRA distributions, and Social Security benefits; business income; unemployment compensation; ordinary dividends; alimony; rental income; and any other taxable income. You then take any allowable deductions, such as self-employment expenses; tuition and fees; moving expenses; and alimony paid.

To get the _modified_ part, you add back in nontaxable Social Security benefits, tax-exempt interest, and foreign income.

If this all sounds way too complicated to figure out, don't fret: When you apply to the Marketplace, it offers detailed assistance to help you determine your MAGI.

Assessing your household income

First, a key definition: Your household includes yourself, your spouse, and your *dependents* — anyone you claim as an exemption on your federal income tax. Obviously, this definition includes children, but it also may include adults who live with you year-round and receive most of their support from you.

Your income level and household size are key factors in determining whether you can expect to qualify for a tax credit when you apply for coverage on the Marketplace. In general, if your income falls within these ranges, you may qualify for tax credits for your coverage in 2014. And within these broad ranges, lower incomes qualify for higher credits.

- ✔ $11,490 to $45,960 for individuals
- ✔ $15,510 to $62,040 for a family of two
- ✔ $19,530 to $78,120 for a family of three
- ✔ $23,550 to $94,200 for a family of four
- ✔ $27,570 to $110,280 for a family of five
- ✔ $31,590 to $126,360 for a family of six
- ✔ $35,610 to $142,440 for a family of seven
- ✔ $39,630 to $158,520 for a family of eight

Beginning in November 2014, new, higher numbers will be in effect for coverage that starts 2015.

Reducing Out-of-Pocket Expenses

A significant financial protection the ACA provides relates to out-of-pocket costs. Whereas limits on these costs didn't exist before the law's passage, as of 2014, the maximum out-of-pocket costs for any insurance plan sold on the Marketplace are $6,350 for an individual plan and $12,700 for a family plan. These numbers will increase each year.

In addition, the ACA requires that insurers selling plans on the Marketplace offer *cost-sharing reduction,* which lowers the out-of-pocket costs you incur when you get medical care. As with the tax credit, your eligibility for this reduction is based on your household size and income. Find your household size in this list; if your household income is lower than the associated amount, you likely qualify for this reduction:

- ✔ $28,725 for an individual
- ✔ $38,775 for two
- ✔ $48,825 for three
- ✔ $58,875 for four
- ✔ $68,925 for five
- ✔ $78,975 for six
- ✔ $89,025 for seven
- ✔ $99,075 for eight

To get the savings, you must enroll in a silver plan, which is a midlevel insurance plan (see Chapter 3). Basically, you get the out-of-pocket benefit of having a gold or platinum plan, but you pay the lower premium of a silver plan.

Considering Tax Implications

The healthcare law makes several changes to taxes that mostly affect individuals with incomes over $200,000, or couples with income over $250,000.

In this section, we explain changes you may notice and discuss whether they're a source of concern or simply something to be aware of.

W-2 reporting

You may notice on your W-2 form that your employer has reported the cost of your group health insurance benefits. This new reporting doesn't affect the taxes you pay. When you file your taxes, you don't report the value of any health insurance benefits on your W-2; no Medicare taxes are withheld on this amount, either.

Medicare taxes

Your Medicare taxes will not increase if you earn less than
$200,000 (or less than $250,000 for a couple filing a joint tax
return). Your earnings that are less than $200,000 (or $250,000
for a couple) will continue to be taxed at 1.45 percent.

If you earn more than $200,000 as an individual taxpayer (or
more than $250,000 as a couple), you will see an increase in the
amount you owe for Medicare taxes. The tax rate on the portion of your earnings above these amounts has increased from
1.45 percent to 2.35 percent. Your employer will continue to
pay the employer's portion of the tax at 1.45 percent on all your
earnings and will withhold the employee portion of the tax.

Investment income tax

If your income is more than $200,000 as an individual taxpayer
or more than $250,000 as a couple, you now pay a 3.8 percent
tax on some of your investment income as a result of the ACA.
Taxpayers with an income of less than $200,000 or $250,000
for a couple filing a joint tax return do not pay higher taxes on
their investment income.

Not all investment income is taxed. The tax applies to interest,
dividends, annuities, royalties, rents, and capital gains that are
subject to income tax. It doesn't include income from Social
Security, pensions, IRA distributions, or qualified IRA annuity
payments.

To figure out the amount of the tax, subtract $200,000 (for an
individual) or $250,000 (for a couple) from your modified
adjusted gross income. Then compare the result with your
net investment income. Multiply the lesser amount by
3.8 percent to get the amount of the tax.

For example, a married couple with a MAGI of $275,000 and a net
investment income of $10,000 would pay $380 in taxes on their
net investment income: $275,000 − $250,000 = $25,000, which
is larger than $10,000 for a tax of $10,000 × 3.8 percent = $380.

Check with the IRS or your tax adviser for additional tax
information.

Flexible spending accounts (FSA)

Some employers offer flexible spending accounts (FSA) that allow you to set aside part of your salary before it's taxed to help pay for some of your medical expenses. If you have an FSA, the most you can now contribute to it is $2,500. Under the ACA, this limit will go up in future years with inflation. And certain over-the-counter medications, such as aspirin or cough syrup, are no longer reimbursed through an FSA unless a doctor prescribes them.

Medical expense deductions

If you itemize your tax deductions, you can deduct only medical expenses that exceed 10 percent (not the previous 7.5 percent) of your adjusted gross income. For example, if your adjusted gross income is $100,000 and your medical expenses are $12,000, you can deduct $2,000 in medical expenses: $12,000 – [$100,000 × 10% or $10,000] = $2,000.

The floor will remain at 7.5 percent through 2016 for persons 65 and older or anyone who is married to a spouse age 65 or older.

New tax on "Cadillac" health plans

Starting in 2018, your insurer will pay a 40 percent tax on the portion of your health benefit premiums that are above $10,200 for individual plans and $27,500 for family plans. The thresholds increase to $11,850 and $30,950 for some younger retirees not eligible for Medicare, as well as people in high-risk occupations. All levels will be indexed to the cost of living. If you're self-employed and you get your insurance through a group health plan, your plan insurer will also have to pay the tax.

You do not directly pay this so-called "Cadillac plan tax" because your insurer or plan sponsor owes the tax. An insurer can be an insurance company, your employer (if it self-funds its insurance plan), or a third party that handles your employer's health plans. Your insurer must determine whether it will pass on the cost of the tax to you or to your employer.

Part II
Impacting Medicare, Small Businesses, and Special Groups

Five Ways the ACA Influences Medicare

- ✔ You may pay less for preventive services.
- ✔ You may pay less for prescription drugs.
- ✔ Your Medicare Advantage plan may improve.
- ✔ You may experience better coordinated care.
- ✔ Medicare waste, fraud, and abuse may decrease.

Check out a helpful article that outlines nine ways to compare Medicare and Medicare Advantage at www.dummies.com/extras/affordablecareact.

In this part . . .

✔ Recognize how the ACA intersects with Medicare, encouraging your healthcare providers to work toward your optimal health by coordinating your care.

✔ Navigate the SHOP Marketplace to select a health plan for small business employees.

✔ Get familiar with important insurance protections for young adults and LGBT households.

✔ Understand your insurance options if you're self-employed, a part-time employee, or unemployed.

✔ Seek the most robust prenatal and pediatric care by taking advantage of key ACA provisions for mothers and children.

Chapter 5

Interacting with Medicare

· ·

In This Chapter

▶ Getting to know some Medicare basics

▶ Paying less for preventive care and prescriptions

▶ Rewarding high-quality providers

▶ Improving your healthcare via greater coordination

▶ Impacting Part D premiums in higher income brackets

▶ Tackling problems such as waste and fraud

· ·

*T*he Affordable Care Act doesn't replace Medicare, but it does influence Medicare in several ways.

If you already have Medicare, you almost certainly don't need health coverage under the ACA. So if it's time for you to enroll in Medicare, you'll sign up for it just as you would if the ACA weren't in place, by visiting www.socialsecurity.gov or calling Social Security at 800-772-1213.

The ACA also doesn't change Medicare's open enrollment period, the time when you can compare different types of coverage in Medicare and change to another plan, if you choose. That period runs from October 15 to December 7 each year.

The ways in which the ACA does change Medicare mostly come into play when you use healthcare services, such as visiting a doctor or paying for a prescription drug.

In this chapter, we first give you a quick rundown of some Medicare fundamentals so we're all speaking the same language. We then outline the key ways in which the ACA and Medicare interact so you can anticipate how your Medicare coverage may differ because of the ACA.

A Medicare Primer

Many people get confused about how Medicare's many options work. Think of a big park. Every path you go down leads to a different section, offering a choice of activities — but whichever path you pick, you're still in the park. The same is true of Medicare. You can choose different kinds of healthcare coverage within the program, and you can choose how you want your medical services delivered — the traditional way or through a private health plan. Whichever you choose, you still have Medicare.

If you're enrolled in Medicare Parts A and B, or even Part A alone, you've got sufficient coverage so you'll face no financial penalties under the ACA. However, if you're enrolled in Part B alone (without Part A), this does not meet the ACA's requirement for "minimum essential coverage." Few people have Part B alone, but if you're in this situation, you should sign up for insurance under the ACA to avoid penalties. (See Chapter 4 for a discussion of the financial consequences of having no healthcare coverage.)

Figuring out Medicare's parts

Medicare has three parts that provide coverage for different types of healthcare:

- ✓ **Part A:** Helps pay the costs when you're a patient in the hospital. (In specific and limited circumstances, Part A may also help cover the costs of care in a skilled nursing facility or hospice, or at-home treatment by a home healthcare team.)

- ✓ **Part B:** Helps pay the costs of doctors' services and using Medicare-approved outpatient services (such as lab tests, screenings, and medical equipment).

- ✓ **Part D:** Helps pay the costs of prescription drugs that you take yourself. (Part A covers medications administered in a hospital; Part B generally covers those administered in a doctor's office.)

There are two ways you can get your Medicare and prescription drug coverage:

✔ **Traditional (or original) Medicare:** This option works the way it has since Medicare began in 1966. When you use a Medicare service, you pay a share of the bill (such as your hospital deductible and typically 20 percent of the cost of outpatient services), and Medicare pays the remainder directly to the provider. This "fee-for-service" system of charges is the same for everybody in traditional Medicare. You can go to any provider in the United States that accepts Medicare patients. Traditional Medicare includes Parts A and B. If you want Part D, you must choose and join a Medicare-approved Part D private drug plan.

✔ **Medicare Advantage (also known as Part C):** This option provides several alternatives to traditional Medicare, each offered through many private insurance plans that Medicare approves and regulates. Medicare gives each plan a set amount of money toward the care of each person enrolled in the plan, regardless of how much healthcare that person uses. You pay what the plan requires for each service.

Each Medicare Advantage plan must provide at least the same services as traditional Medicare but may offer extra benefits. Costs and benefits vary a great deal among plans. Some enrollees pay less than they would in traditional Medicare, and others pay more. You must be enrolled in both Medicare Part A and Part B to join a Medicare Advantage plan. Most plans charge a monthly premium (in addition to the Part B premium), but depending on where you live, you may find plans that don't. Most Medicare Advantage plans also include Part D, so you get your health and prescription drug coverage in one plan. Also, you can't use a Medigap supplemental policy to limit your costs if you're enrolled in a Medicare Advantage plan. But all Advantage plans set an annual limit on what you pay out of pocket. These are important distinctions between original Medicare and Medicare Advantage plans.

Here, briefly, are the main features of different types of Medicare Advantage plans:

• *Health Maintenance Organizations (HMOs)* operate in local areas (counties and sometimes zip codes). You can typically go only to the doctors and hospitals within the plan's provider network (except in emergencies or for urgently needed care), and you must go through a primary-care physician to see specialists.

- *Preferred Provider Organizations (PPOs)* may operate locally (in counties) or regionally (in part of a state or groups of adjacent states). They have provider networks but allow you to go to doctors and hospitals outside the network for a higher copayment and to see specialists without a referral.

- *Private Fee-for-Service (PFFS)* plans are mostly required by law to establish contracts with doctors, hospitals, and other providers. You must go to your plan's specified providers or pay more to go out of its network, except in emergencies. In the case of some rural PFFS plans that are not required to have formal contracts with providers, check to see how your preferred doctors and hospitals would work with the plan you're considering.

- *Medicare Medical Savings Accounts (MSAs)* deposit a portion of the money they receive from Medicare into a personal health savings account that you set up. At the same time, you participate in a high deductible Medicare Advantage plan, which begins to cover your healthcare costs only after you meet a high yearly deductible, which varies by plan. You pay for medical services (from any providers of your choice) out of the MSA. When the money is exhausted, you pay 100 percent out of pocket until you've met your deductible. After your expenses meet that limit, the plan pays 100 percent of your costs until the end of the year. You can roll over any money left in your medical savings account into the following year, and it's yours to keep if you don't re-enroll in the plan. You must file tax forms on your MSA withdrawals and pay tax on any expenses that don't count as qualified medical expenses. Note, though, that MSAs are now available in very few places.

- *Special Needs Plans (SNPs)* are either HMOs or PPOs. Each SNP serves the needs of one special category of Medicare beneficiaries — people who receive both Medicare and Medicaid, or people who live in institutions (such as nursing homes), or people who have at least one chronic or disabling condition (such as diabetes, congestive heart failure, mental illness, or HIV/AIDS). Some SNPs offer the services of care managers to coordinate enrollees' healthcare, financial, and community needs. SNPs aren't available in all areas of the country.

You can compare the details of traditional Medicare and specific private health plans available in your area by using Medicare's online health plan finder tool, which you access at `www.medicare.gov/find-a-plan/questions/home.aspx`.

Getting Part D prescription drug coverage

Part D drug coverage works through private plans, in two ways. You can choose a stand-alone plan that covers only prescription drugs, or you can choose a Medicare Advantage private health plan that combines medical benefits and prescription drug coverage in one package. Which type you can select depends on how you receive your medical benefits:

✔ You can choose a stand-alone drug plan if you're enrolled in:

  • Traditional Medicare

  • A Medicare medical savings account

  • A private fee-for-service plan that does not cover drugs

✔ You can choose a Medicare private health plan (HMO, PPO, PFFS, or SNP) that combines medical care and prescription drug coverage in its benefit package.

You cannot be enrolled in a stand-alone drug plan at the same time you're in a Medicare HMO or PPO, even if that plan doesn't cover drugs.

Distinguishing Medigap and Medicare Advantage plans

These two types of insurance are very different, although both are options for people with Medicare. Technically, only Medigap counts as *Medicare supplemental insurance* — in fact, that's its formal name — but Medicare Advantage plans may provide some extra benefits.

Only people enrolled in traditional Medicare can use Medigap. It's not a government-run program — it's private insurance you can purchase to cover some or most of your out-of-pocket expenses in traditional Medicare. These expenses may include Part B costs, like the 20 percent you'd otherwise pay for physician visits and other outpatient services, the Part A hospital deductible ($1,216 in 2014 for each hospital benefit period), most of the cost of medical emergencies abroad, and certain other outlays, depending on which kind of policy you choose. Each of the ten types of Medigap policies is standardized by law — meaning the benefits of each are the same, regardless of which insurer sells it. But insurers still charge widely different premiums, so it pays to shop around.

If you're 65 or older, it's best to buy Medigap at a time when you have full federal protections, which prohibit insurers from denying coverage or charging higher premiums based on past or present health issues. Typically, this time frame is within six months of enrolling in Medicare Part B or within two months of losing primary health coverage from an employer or union. If you have Medicare under age 65 because of disability, these federal rules do not apply to you, but some states provide similar protections.

If you enroll in a Medicare Advantage health plan, you cannot use a Medigap policy to pay out-of-pocket expenses under that health plan, and it is illegal for an insurer to sell you a Medigap policy. If you stay in traditional Medicare, you need to join a separate Part D plan to get prescription drug coverage and pay an extra premium for it. Medigap also doesn't cover out-of-pocket drug expenses under Medicare Part D.

Comparing and choosing plans

When deciding whether to buy a Medigap policy to cover expenses in traditional Medicare or enroll in a Medicare Advantage plan, it's important to look at the details of each plan available to you, to find the one that best suits your needs and pocketbook. Medicare has online programs to help you make these comparisons:

✔ **Medigap policies:** Visit the Medigap Policy finder at www.medicare.gov/find-a-plan/questions/medigap-home.aspx. Enter your zip code and follow the instructions. You will see a chart showing all the policies (each labeled with a different letter of the alphabet) available in your area. Clicking on the name of any policy brings up full information for that policy. To see which insurers sell the policy, click on View Companies on the right side of the chart. You'll see contact information for the companies and can contact them for a premium quote.

If you have Medicare because of disability: Medigap policies aren't always available to beneficiaries younger than age 65 and may cost more, depending on which state you live in. To see the situation in your own area, first go to the Medigap Policy finder at www.medicare. gov/find-a-plan/questions/medigap-home.aspx and enter your zip code. Click on the link marked Show Only Policies Available to People under Age 65, at the top of the chart that lists all policies. If any appear, click on those for details and then click on View Companies.

✓ **Medicare Advantage plans:** Visit the Medicare plan finder at www.medicare.gov/find-a-plan/questions/ home.aspx. Enter your zip code and follow the instructions. Eventually, you will see a list of about ten health plans. To see the full list of plans available in your area, click on View 20 or View 50, at the top of the list. This page provides broad information such as premiums, whether the plans cover prescription drugs, and how Medicare has rated each plan for its quality according to a range of measures (such as customer service) on a scale of one to five stars. To see details of each plan's costs and benefits, click on the name of the plan.

If you have Medicare because of disability: Medicare Advantage plans are available to beneficiaries under age 65, with one exception. You generally cannot enroll in any of these plans if you already have end-stage renal disease, defined as needing regular dialysis or a kidney transplant.

Medicare Changes under the ACA

With the basics of Medicare under your belt, you're now ready to read about how the ACA improves the healthcare you receive as a Medicare enrollee and reduces the money you're paying out of pocket for those services.

Paying less for preventive services

If you have Medicare, you can work with your doctor on a prevention plan to keep you as healthy as possible. Under the ACA, you are entitled to the following preventive benefits at no cost to you.

- ✔ A yearly wellness visit. This is a Medicare Part B service and can be provided by a physician, physician assistant, nurse practitioner, or clinical nurse specialist as well as other types of professionals. The annual wellness visit is specifically designed to identify certain risk factors, provide personalized health advice, and refer patients for additional preventive services or interventions (which Medicare may or may not pay for). During this visit, your care provider will develop a personalized prevention plan tailored to your needs and health goals. This plan can be updated on subsequent annual visits.

- ✔ Screenings to prevent and detect health problems, including screenings for diabetes, high cholesterol, and certain cancers. Mammograms and colonoscopies, for example, are covered at no cost to you. But related procedures may have a cost — for instance, if the doctor finds and biopsies a polyp during a routine colonoscopy.

- ✔ Recommended vaccines to help prevent health problems.

The yearly wellness visit is different than a physical; a physical is a more extensive exam. You may choose to have a physical at another visit with your doctor, but Medicare will not pay for this service. If you have a Medicare Advantage plan, ask whether your plan pays for a yearly physical exam; if it doesn't, you will be responsible for payment. To view what a yearly wellness visit includes, go to www.medicare.gov/coverage/preventive-visit-and-yearly-wellness-exams.html.

If you're new to Medicare, you should know that the program covers a one-time free Welcome to Medicare physical exam, which is available during the first 12 months of your enrollment. This benefit is designed to establish a personalized prevention plan for you as early as possible, which can be developed during annual wellness visits in subsequent years. For this reason, the wellness visit is not available during your first year in Medicare.

Most Medicare Advantage plans offer Medicare-covered preventive services with no deductibles and copayments. The ACA doesn't require Medicare Advantage plans to offer preventive services free of charge. If you have a Medicare Advantage plan, check with your plan to confirm the deductibles and copayments for preventive services, if any.

The ACA's provision for preventive services at no cost to you is having a significant financial impact on Medicare participants. In 2013, more than 25 million people with traditional Medicare received at least one free preventive service, such as an annual wellness visit or mammogram.

Closing the prescription drug coverage gap

Prescription drug coverage plays a vital role in the health and financial security of older and disabled adults. For many people who have Medicare, this ACA provision is a biggie. If you have prescription drug coverage under Medicare Part D and you fall into the coverage gap known as the *doughnut hole,* you should see greatly reduced out-of-pocket drug costs in the future because of the ACA. Instead of paying 100 percent of the cost of your drugs in the gap (which happened until 2011), you now get discounts on brand-name and generic prescription drugs, and these discounts will continue to increase until 2020, when the doughnut hole will disappear.

However, everyone with Medicare Part D will still have out-of-pocket costs for premiums and copayments, just like you do now before you reach the doughnut hole. You will still be responsible for paying your premiums and deductible as well as 25 percent of your prescription drug costs until you reach catastrophic coverage.

Not sure what the doughnut hole is? It's a gap in coverage that occurs after the total cost of your drugs (what you've paid and what your plan has paid) reaches a certain dollar limit in any given year. If your costs exceed that amount, you're in the coverage gap, which continues until you've spent a certain amount out of pocket since the beginning of the year ($4,550 in 2014). At that point, you qualify for *catastrophic coverage*, under which you pay no more than 5 percent of the cost of your drugs until the end of the year.

The doughnut hole discounts created by the ACA come partly from the drug manufacturers (in the case of brand-name drugs) and partly from the federal government (for generic drugs).

The discounts are calculated automatically when you purchase the drug from a pharmacy. You don't need to fill out any additional paperwork or apply to any program to receive them. Another bit of good news: The discounts you receive for brand-name drugs don't prolong your stay in the doughnut hole. Their value counts toward the out-of-pocket limit that gets you out of the gap, even though you don't actually pay them.

As of late 2013, more than 7 million seniors and people with disabilities on Medicare had already saved nearly $9 billion on prescription drugs thanks to the ACA, according to data released by the Centers for Medicare & Medicaid Services. Those savings will balloon as the coverage gap continues to close.

AARP provides an online calculator at www.aarp.org/ doughnuthole that can help you figure out if and when you might hit the coverage gap. This tool also provides suggestions for alternative medications that you can discuss with your doctors. The lower-cost medications might help you avoid the coverage gap entirely.

Improving Medicare Advantage plans

The ACA contains provisions intended to improve how Medicare Advantage plans work. As we explain earlier in the chapter (see "Figuring out Medicare's four parts"), Medicare Advantage plans are an alternative to traditional Medicare. These plans are offered by private insurance companies and pay for the same healthcare services as traditional Medicare, but they also may charge less and pay for additional healthcare services that traditional Medicare doesn't cover. With most Medicare Advantage plans, you need to see the doctors and use the hospitals that are part of the plan's network.

The ACA affects Medicare Advantage plans in three key ways:

✔ **Rewarding high-quality care:** Medicare rates each Medicare Advantage plan by compiling information gleaned from the plans themselves, participant satisfaction surveys, and healthcare providers. The ratings, which are awarded each fall (and can change from year to year), are on a five-star basis: a low-quality plan may receive only one star, whereas the highest-quality plans get five. Under the ACA, Medicare Advantage plans that rate at least three out of five stars receive bonus payments for providing better-quality care. Plans that receive fewer than three stars for three years in a row are terminated from Medicare.

You can review your plan's rating on Medicare's website at www.medicare.gov, or call Medicare at 800-633-4227.

✔ **Limiting administrative costs:** The law requires that plans limit how much they spend each year on administrative costs. For each dollar you pay in premiums, your Medicare Advantage plan must spend at least 85 cents on healthcare costs.

✔ **Reducing federal payments:** Before the ACA, Medicare was overpaying the private companies that offer Medicare Advantage plans. This means that these plans cost the Medicare program more than traditional Medicare. The law gradually eliminates the overpayments, so that eventually Medicare's payments to the plans will be more in line with traditional Medicare. This could result in some plans dropping out of Medicare in some areas.

Every year, even before the Affordable Care Act, insurance companies that offered Medicare Advantage plans made decisions about what they would cover, what they would charge, and whether they will continue to provide service in an area. Each insurance company will continue to make these same business decisions.

You always have the option to stay with your current plan or switch to a new one during Medicare's open enrollment period, which takes place from October 15 to December 7. You must receive a notice from your insurance company in September telling you what changes, if any, will take place in your Medicare plan for the upcoming plan year. You can then compare your options and make a well-informed decision. You can keep your plan, switch to another, or opt for traditional Medicare. If you have questions about the notice, you can contact your Medicare Advantage plan directly, or you can call Medicare at 800-633-4227.

Coordinating your care

The ACA encourages greater coordination among healthcare providers, to promote better care for patients and reduce costs related to duplicated care. For example, the law provides for the creation of *accountable care organizations* (ACOs) in the traditional Medicare program. These are networks of doctors, hospitals, and other healthcare providers who agree to work together to coordinate Medicare patient care.

ACOs are designed to combat the "silo" approach to healthcare, in which a Medicare patient moves from provider to provider seeking care, but the patient's information doesn't necessarily move with him. The patient then is forced to try to link together various types of care to achieve better health. The ACO network approach, in contrast, pays the participating healthcare providers for coordinating the patient's care. A primary care physician, specialists, home health care agencies, hospitals, and any other providers all have access to a network patient's medical information and work together as a team to plan that individual's care.

As a Medicare patient, you should keep in mind a couple key points about this new approach:

- ✔ If your primary care physician, specialists, or other providers participate in an ACO, you're not limited to working only with them. You have the right to seek care outside that network of providers, if you choose.

- ✔ If your healthcare providers participate in an ACO, they must tell you. You decide whether to allow network providers to share your healthcare information. If you prefer that your information *not* be shared among your doctor, specialists, and hospital, you have the right to say no.

If you have questions about how participating in an ACO may impact your care, or if you're concerned about privacy issues when your healthcare providers share your medical records, talk to your doctor or other providers, or contact Medicare at 800-633-4227.

Preparing for premium changes if your income is high

The ACA includes an important change in Medicare Part D premiums for people with higher incomes. Since 2007, people have paid higher premiums for Part B if their modified adjusted gross income (MAGI), as reported on their latest tax returns, is above a certain level: $85,000 for a single person and $170,000 for married couples filing joint tax returns.

Income-related premiums now also apply to people who have Part D prescription drug coverage. The MAGI levels are the same as for Part B, and both will stay the same until 2020. It's important to know, though, that if you're required to pay these surcharges but your income suddenly drops due to a specified "life-changing event" — such as retirement, loss of earnings, marriage, or divorce — you should apply immediately to Social Security for an adjustment.

Be aware that a short-term increase in income — for example, from the sale of a house or a distribution from a tax-deferred account such as an IRA or a 401K — may increase your MAGI enough to require surcharges on your Part B and Part D premiums for that particular year.

Fighting waste, fraud, and abuse

The ACA contains provisions that specifically tackle waste, fraud, and abuse in the Medicare system. For example:

- ✔ The law encourages healthcare providers to work together to reduce duplicate and unnecessary services while simultaneously improving patient care; see the earlier section "Coordinating your care."

- ✔ Insurance companies that provide Medicare Advantage plans must take training that addresses how to reduce waste.

✔ The law allows federal law enforcement agencies faster and better access to data that help them quickly identify and halt instances of fraud.

✔ The ACA puts in place more tools to screen healthcare providers who participate in Medicare and to catch providers who fraudulently bill the program. Also, money is available to reward Medicare beneficiaries who report incidents that prove to be fraudulent.

In taking these steps, the ACA aims to significantly reduce improper payments and inappropriate costs associated with Medicare, to help ensure that the program is funded for years to come.

Chapter 6

Shopping for Plans as a Small Business Owner

In This Chapter

▶ Figuring out what the ACA requires for your business

▶ Understanding your new protections

▶ Preparing to SHOP for plan options

▶ Helping your employees review your selection

*F*inding and keeping good health insurance coverage has been especially challenging for small businesses. Before the ACA, if one worker got sick, premiums for everyone could go up a lot — often making coverage unaffordable for the owners and their workers. And these high costs made it harder to offer good benefits.

For these reasons, the ACA has rules specifically for coverage sold to small business owners. In this chapter, we introduce you to the new rules so that if you own a small business — or work for a small business — you have the basic information you need to understand your health insurance options and anticipate how they're changing.

This chapter is by no means the final word on what you can do as a small business owner to take advantage of the ACA's provisions. For additional information and support as you determine your best options, be sure to visit www.healthcare.gov and click on the "Small Businesses" tab; use the information and tools available from the U.S. Small Business Administration (http://www.sba.gov/healthcare); and work with a licensed insurance broker or agent if the process seems overwhelming.

Determining Whether You Need to Provide Coverage

Before we get into the discussion of how the ACA affects small business coverage options, we want to address a fundamental question: Does the healthcare law require businesses to provide coverage to their employees? The answer is no. Starting in 2015, however, a large business must provide health coverage or face financial tax penalties.

✔ **Small businesses:** About 96 percent of all businesses in the United States are categorized as small businesses — those with 50 or fewer full-time equivalent employees. These businesses have never been required to provide health insurance and still aren't required to do so under the ACA.

Notice the phrase *full-time equivalent.* As a business owner, you may employ only part-time workers, so you need to determine how many full-time equivalent employees you have, based on the number of hours worked. See the nearby sidebar on this topic to grasp how the IRS determines the number of full-time equivalent employees you have working for your business.

Although small businesses aren't required to offer coverage, they may choose to tap into the resources the SHOP (Small Business Health Options Program) Marketplace (also called the *exchange*) provides so that they can pool their purchasing power. We discuss this new opportunity in the upcoming section "Navigating the SHOP Marketplace."

✔ **Large businesses:** As mentioned, large businesses must provide health coverage or face financial tax penalties starting in 2015. This provision applies to businesses that have 50 or more full-time equivalent employees (see the nearby sidebar for an explanation of this term). The vast majority of large businesses in the United States were already offering health coverage before the ACA, so this provision doesn't necessarily have a huge impact on most big companies.

However, this provision has a second layer: Large companies must provide insurance coverage that meets two standards:

Full-time equivalent employees

Say you're a business owner and you employ 100 part-time people. Are you a small business or a large business? Which ACA regulations apply to you?

To determine the answer, you need to know how many *full-time equivalent* (FTE) employees you have. All part-time workers are counted in your FTE calculations, but seasonal workers generally are not. (If a seasonal worker is employed for more than 120 days during the year in question, you do count that person toward your FTE calculations.) Business owners and their family members generally aren't included in the calculations either.

Per the IRS, you determine your FTE number by adding up the total hours of service that your employees have been paid for during the year in question. (For a full-time employee, the number is capped at 2,080.) You divide that amount by 2,080 and (if necessary) round the result to the next-lowest whole number.

For example, say that you have 62 part-time employees. In a given year, you pay them for a total of 74,400 service hours. You divide that number by 2,080 to find out that you have 35 FTE employees, which means that you fall into the category of a small business for purposes of the ACA.

- *Affordability:* The employee's share of the premium costs for the lowest-cost plan offered by the employer (to cover the employee only, not that person's family) cannot equal more than 9.5 percent of that person's annual household income. If the employer's plan costs more than this amount, the ACA doesn't consider the plan to be affordable.

- *Minimum value:* The ACA states that a large company's health plan has minimum value if it pays at least 60 percent of the costs of covered services.

A large business offering coverage that doesn't meet both criteria with the insurance it offers to its employees (or that doesn't offer any coverage) may face a financial tax penalty as of 2015. This *Employer Shared Responsibility Payment* takes two forms:

- *No coverage:* If the company doesn't offer its employees any health coverage, each year it will owe a fee (currently $2,000) per full-time equivalent employee, excluding the first 30 employees. The fee will increase each year.

- *Insufficient coverage:* If the company offers a health plan that is subpar per either of the two criteria the ACA has set, each year it will owe a fee (currently $3,000) per full-time equivalent employee if one or more employees gets subsidies in the Health Insurance Marketplace (see Chapter 2).

Currently, large businesses aren't eligible for coverage in a SHOP Marketplace. But the ACA provides that these companies may gain access in 2017 to the SHOP Marketplace if their state chooses to do so.

✓ **Self-employed business owners:** Under the ACA, a self-employed business owner who has no employees is responsible for securing health insurance coverage (or securing an exemption from needing to do so) the same way any other individual is responsible. In other words, self-employed people are covered by the ACA's *individual mandate* to enroll in a health plan.

If you are self-employed with no employees, you need to apply to the Health Insurance Marketplace as an individual rather than as a business to SHOP.

In Chapter 4, we list the groups of people who may secure an exemption from the responsibility to have health insurance. We also discuss the ways in which the ACA is designed to help individuals with lower incomes afford paying for healthcare premiums by shopping on the Health Insurance Marketplace.

If you're self-employed and you don't currently have health coverage, Chapter 2 walks you through the process of applying to the Health Insurance Marketplace so you can peruse your plan options and get an idea of the financial help that may be available.

Recognizing Small Business Protections under the ACA

If you read only the first section of this chapter, you may think that the ACA stands to have a greater impact on individuals and large businesses than it does on small businesses. Not so. Small businesses may feel a significant impact from the ACA, and the overall result should be positive.

According to estimates from the Employee Benefit Research Institute, about half of the people in the United States who were uninsured prior to the passage of the ACA were either self-employed or worked for small businesses. Kaiser Family Foundation research shows that only about one-quarter of small businesses offer healthcare coverage.

The ACA tries to tackle these issues in a couple ways. One way is by helping small business owners combine their purchasing power through the SHOP Marketplace; we discuss this topic in the next section. The other way is by providing small businesses with key protections that didn't exist previously. These protections mirror some of the individual protections the ACA established, which we explain in Chapter 1. Here are the biggies:

✔ **Premium controls:** Insurance plans can no longer charge small businesses more because they have employees with health conditions like diabetes, hypertension, or cancer. If one or more of your employees has an illness or chronic condition that's likely to involve lengthy, expensive medical treatment, you (and that employee) won't be punished for it by watching your premiums skyrocket.

As we explain in Chapter 1, insurers can now take into account only four factors when they establish premium rates:

- Age

- Geographic location

- Tobacco use

- Individual versus family coverage

✔ **Gender equitable coverage:** Insurance plans also can't charge more for businesses that employ more women than men. In the past, insurers often did charge more to provide coverage to women because women historically have used more medical services than men.

✔ **Essential health benefits:** All new insurance plans, including plans that small businesses may opt into via the SHOP Marketplace (see the next section), are required to cover a core set of benefits, including doctor visits, hospitalizations, emergency room care, maternity care, pediatric care, and prescriptions. Check out the complete list of essential health benefits in Chapter 3.

Navigating the SHOP Marketplace

The ACA gives small business a new way to shop for health coverage. If you're a business owner with between 2 and 50 full-time equivalent employees, you can now join with other small businesses in your state to get health insurance for your employees. (If you're the only full-time employee of the business, some states will allow you to be treated as a group of one, or you can access the Marketplace as an individual and possibly qualify for cost savings, as we discuss in Chapter 4.) You should have many more options than you previously did.

Business owners can shop for health insurance plans for employees using their state's online SHOP Marketplace. (We explain the basics of navigating the Marketplace in Chapter 2.) A business owner can choose what plan to offer to employees and determine what to pay toward employee premiums. Then the employees can go online and sign up — or not (see the section "Helping Your Employees Sign Up," later in this chapter).

Creating an online account

Each state has a SHOP Marketplace. To use a specific SHOP, you must have an office or work site in that state. To get started, you can visit www.healthcare.gov/marketplace/shop and click on "Apply Now." Click the link "Set up a Marketplace account online." You're asked to provide basic information about yourself, create a user name and password, and answer some security questions. You then receive an e-mail asking you to confirm that you've applied, and you're on your way. You need to have an account created for your business before you can choose a plan and get employees signed up.

If you prefer to speak with a Marketplace customer service representative, you can call 800-706-7893 (TTY: 1-800-706-7915) Monday through Friday from 9 a.m. until 7 p.m. ET.

This system, which is in its infancy as of this writing, is designed to reduce a business owner's paperwork and administrative costs. In addition, the goal is to provide greater leverage for driving down insurance costs by grouping coverage purchases for many small businesses within each state. SHOP gives smaller employers more buying power: They pool their risk and have a better selection of plans at a lower cost. According to the U.S. Small Business Administration, before the ACA, small businesses paid an average of 18 percent more than larger businesses for their health insurance. The new provisions are designed to level the playing field.

Choosing the right plan for your business

As we note earlier in the chapter, small business owners aren't required to offer their employees health coverage. But if you do, the SHOP Marketplace is an easy way to search for coverage and compare plans and costs.

In Chapter 2, we explain the Summary of Benefits and Coverage (SBC) that insurers are now required to provide for each private health plan, whether offered through an employer or on the Marketplace. The SBC is a standard form that must be completed in easily understood language so that everyone perusing options on the Marketplace, including small business owners, can easily do an apples-to-apples comparison among plan options.

The SHOP Marketplace (like the general Marketplace for individuals) offers plans in four metal categories: bronze, silver, gold, and platinum. The plan levels do *not* represent the quality of the health coverage you receive. Instead, the metals represent various levels of coverage you receive and the relative generosity of what the plan pays on average. A bronze plan has the lowest premiums and highest out-of-pocket costs, so it offers lower monthly payments but the greatest risk if you have a serious medical issue. A platinum plan is at the other end of the spectrum: It has the highest premiums but lowest out-of-pocket costs, so the monthly financial commitment is high, but the risk is lower when medical issues arise.

With that said, each plan in the SHOP Marketplace is unique, so don't look *solely* at cost when making comparisons. You want to judge each plan based on its full scope of benefits as well. Depending on your employees' needs, the lowest-cost plans may not give the best overall value.

Refer to Chapter 3 for a more thorough discussion of the four metal plan categories, as well as a look at catastrophic plans. If you need a refresher on out-of-pocket costs such as deductibles and copayments, flip to Chapter 4.

Working with a broker or agent

If you're a small business owner who has been providing insurance coverage to your employees, chances are good that you've previously worked with an insurance broker or agent to compare your options and enroll in a plan. The ACA doesn't require you to change your way of doing business: If you prefer to continue to work with your broker or agent and to avoid interaction with the SHOP Marketplace, that's your choice. However, SHOP well may offer lower-cost options for your consideration, *and it's the only place you can qualify for tax credits.* If the idea of shopping for a plan on your own intimidates you, ask a licensed broker or agent to work with you to review plans on your SHOP Marketplace. This person can help you enroll in a plan offered on SHOP and can then help your employees enroll for coverage.

While SHOP is open now to small businesses with up to 50 full-time equivalent employees, this Marketplace will be extended in the future so that larger businesses may use it as well. In 2016, SHOP is slated to accommodate businesses with up to 100 full-time equivalent employees. In 2017, states will have the option to let larger businesses have access, as well.

If you're a small business owner and you choose to enroll in a SHOP Marketplace plan, you must offer plan coverage to all your full-time employees. In other words, you can't enroll and then get coverage only for yourself and a select few other people. In fact, in most states, if you sign up outside the annual open enrollment period, at least 70 percent of your employees must choose to participate in the coverage you've selected for coverage to begin. The best way to find out what your state requires is to submit a SHOP Marketplace application on www.healthcare.gov/marketplace/shop.

Taking advantage of tax credits

In addition to tapping into cost savings and the protections the ACA offers, small businesses may be eligible for a tax credit that makes the cost of offering employees coverage more affordable.

Tax credits are available to a business that meets these criteria:

- ✔ It employs up to 25 full-time equivalent people.

- ✔ Its employees' average wages are $50,000 or less.

- ✔ The business covers at least half the cost of healthcare coverage for each individual employee. (If employees have family plans, that additional cost isn't considered.)

- ✔ The business uses the SHOP Marketplace. Plans purchased through a broker or agent outside of SHOP don't qualify.

The credit is available for two consecutive years and covers up to half of the employer contribution toward employee premiums, or for a nonprofit (tax-exempt) organization, the credits cover up to 35 percent. The amount of the credit works on a sliding scale, so smaller businesses receive bigger credits.

If you receive a credit for a portion of the premiums you pay, you can still deduct as a business expenses the remainder of the employee premiums that you pay. And if you don't owe any taxes during the year in which you receive the credit, you can apply it to another tax year. For a nonprofit organization, it may be possible to receive the credit in the form of a refund.

To claim this credit, businesses use IRS Form 8941. Visit `www.irs.gov/pub/irs-pdf/i8941.pdf` to view or print the form.

Helping Your Employees Sign Up

If you opt to offer your employees coverage through SHOP, they can sign up for coverage online through the SHOP Marketplace. During your application process, you're asked to provide SHOP with a roster of your employees. After you select a plan, either you or the Marketplace can notify your employees and tell them how to sign up.

You need to decide on the initial employee enrollment period. If you have few employees, you may want to make the window fairly small because it shouldn't take long to help each employee get the information he or she needs. But if you have close to 50 employees, you want to build in enough time to make sure everyone has opportunities to ask questions, do research, and find out the necessary information to make an informed decision.

After the notification goes out to employees, they need to take the following steps on the Marketplace to enroll:

1. **Confirm the information you provided to SHOP.** This information includes the employee name, date of birth, and Social Security number.

2. **Provide additional information.** An employee supplies an address, contact preferences, information about tobacco use (which affects premium rates), and whether any dependents need coverage. This information is needed so the Marketplace can get specific about each person's cost to enroll in the plan you selected.

3. **Consider the plan costs and benefits.** Costs include monthly premiums, as well as out-of-pocket expenses such as deductibles and copays. Benefits must include all the essential health benefits we outline in Chapter 3 and may include others, as well.

If an employee wants to enroll, he enrolls. He then can print a summary of the coverage the plan offers.

Keep in mind, however, that coverage doesn't begin for that employee on the day he signs up. At the end of the enrollment period you've designated, you must review the number of people who have accepted plan coverage, which includes dependents. If enough people have signed up to satisfy your state's requirements (which for many states means 70 percent of your employees are participating), you can proceed with enrollment.

Some states are offering more flexibility than others with SHOP plan options. For example, you may be able to let your employees choose among several plans that are at the same metal level (such as silver or gold; see Chapter 3) or among plans offered by a specific insurer. It's possible you may even be able to offer employees a specific level of financial help based on a benchmark plan that you select, and they can apply that amount to any plan they prefer. Check out your state SHOP website or work with an insurance agent or broker to find out what options are available in your state.

Chapter 7

Considering Special Circumstances

● ●

In This Chapter

▶ Extending coverage options for young adults

▶ Providing greater protections for LGBT households

▶ Considering people who are self-employed, work part time, and are unemployed

▶ Helping parents-to-be and new parents tap into new benefits

● ●

*C*hances are, you're reading this chapter because you count yourself part of a group of people whose healthcare coverage may be impacted in unique ways by the Affordable Care Act. If you're a student or young adult; part of a LGBT household; self-employed, a part-time employee, or unemployed; or a parent-to-be or new parent, this chapter contains some details about the healthcare law that apply specifically to you.

Providing for Young Adults

The ACA requires every American (including children) to have health coverage, but the law recognizes that young adults aren't always in the same employment situations as older adults. Many young people attend college or trade schools and work, at most, part-time jobs while they do so. Others get their first employment experience by working one or more part-time jobs that don't offer coverage.

For these reasons, everyone up to the age of 26 can now remain on (or be added to) a parent's family insurance policies — even if a young adult is married, financially independent, living in a separate location, and/or employed by a company that offers insurance coverage.

If you're the parent of a student or another young adult under the age of 26 and you have family coverage through an employer, keep in mind that your current health plan may charge more for each child you cover. Also note that employers are not required to offer family plan coverage options. Before you make any decisions, check with your employer for the details about adding your adult child to your family plan.

If you're a parent who purchases health coverage through the Health Insurance Marketplace (see Chapter 2), you can sign up directly in the Marketplace to put your adult child on your plan. Again, the premiums you pay may increase to provide this additional coverage.

What about young adults for whom enrolling in a parent's family plan isn't an option? If you can't be covered under your parent's family plan and your employer doesn't offer coverage, you can shop in the Marketplace and tap into the same financial support available to other adults who meet income qualifications (see Chapter 4), such as tax credits that partially offset premium costs. Young adults also can choose among various types of plans that provide different ways to share costs (including premiums and out-of-pocket costs such as deductibles, coinsurance, and copayments) between the insurer and the insured; see Chapter 3 for an explanation of the bronze, silver, gold, and platinum plans on the Marketplace.

In addition, young people up to the age of 30 may choose to forego one of the "metal" plans (see Chapter 3) and enroll instead in a *catastrophic plan,* which has a lower premium but entails significant out-of-pocket expenses if that person requires medical care. Essentially, catastrophic plans are bare bones; they offer protection only in worst-case situations when the insured is badly hurt or seriously ill and requires substantial care. Someone who chooses the catastrophic plan option cannot take advantage of federal government financial subsidies that are available on other Marketplace plans for people whose incomes are below financial thresholds. In other words, the price for catastrophic coverage is not based on your income. The monthly premium is likely lower than what you may pay for coverage through a different type of plan, though the total out-of-pocket costs may not be. And it isn't subject to any tax credits or subsidies.

As we note in Chapter 3, catastrophic plans aren't available for purchase by most people older than age 30 because they're so risky; for example, if you get into an accident or become seriously ill, you can quickly run up thousands of dollars of medical debt before any health coverage kicks in. The only adults over 30 who can buy catastrophic coverage are ones for whom a bronze plan would cost more than 8 percent of their income. In Chapter 4, we explain that the ACA gives certain people exemptions to the requirement of health coverage. The hardship exemption applies to people who have very low incomes or who are otherwise in extremely difficult financial situations and can't afford more comprehensive health insurance.

Supporting LGBT Households

The passage of the ACA, the June 2013 Supreme Court decision that overturned part of the federal Defense of Marriage Act (DOMA), and other recent developments have combined to offer substantial and unprecedented protections for members of the lesbian, gay, bisexual, and transgender (LGBT) community. Here's how:

- ✔ **ACA protections:** Before the passage of the ACA, insurance companies could (and sometimes did) discriminate against individuals, couples, and families based on gender identity and sexual orientation. Companies could legally deny someone coverage because of positive HIV status, for example, or could charge more for a policy because of supposed risk affiliated with sexual orientation.

  The significant patient rights and protections the ACA affords, which we outline in Chapter 1, extend to every American. No one can be denied insurance coverage, face financial penalties in the form of higher premiums, or be subject to benefit exclusions based on gender, gender identity, or sexual orientation.

- ✔ **DOMA implications:** As of 2013, same-sex marriages are recognized for federal benefit purposes. As a result, same-sex couples who are legally married can shop for healthcare coverage in the Marketplace and can apply jointly for federal financial subsidies if their household income qualifies them for assistance (see Chapter 4). The subsidies that offset some of the cost of healthcare premiums are in the form of tax credits, and a married couple can qualify for them even if the state they live in doesn't currently recognize same-sex marriage.

Couples in civil unions or domestic partnerships can also benefit from Marketplace tax credits if their income qualifies them, but they apply for such credits as individuals instead of applying jointly. They then apply any credits they receive to the purchase of a family policy, if needed.

✓ **Changes to Medicaid and CHIP:** In Chapter 1, we explain the state-run Medicaid program and the Child Health Insurance Program (CHIP), which provide healthcare support to low-income individuals and their children. If you or your children are approved for coverage through either program, you most likely meet the ACA's individual mandate: the requirement that every American secure insurance coverage or face possible financial penalties.

Both programs receive federal financial support. Therefore, the Supreme Court's overturning of DOMA impacts these programs as well. Specifically, state governments are now able to recognize same-sex marriages when calculating household income for determining program eligibility. For details about your state's Medicaid and CHIP policies related to same-sex marriages and partnerships, contact your state's programs directly. Start by visiting http://www.medicaid.gov/ and using the "Medicaid Moving Forward" tool on the home page to locate your state's policies.

✓ **Legal protections:** Recent policies issued by the U.S. Department of Health and Human Services have also added protections for the LGBT community in healthcare settings. Some of the biggest protections include the following:

- Hospitals that receive federal funding (such as through Medicare and Medicaid) can no longer prohibit same-sex partner visitation. Same-sex partners must receive the same visitation privileges as spouses.

- The same is true in long-term care settings such as nursing homes, which must treat same-sex partners the same as other spouses in their visitation policies.

- Facilities that receive federal funds also must comply with regulations that give patients the right to determine who should make decisions about their care. Hospitals and nursing homes cannot prohibit same-sex spouses or partners from being named as proxies of *advanced directives:* any documents, such as living wills, that specify the patient's healthcare choices.

If you're part of an LGBT household and you don't have insurance coverage for yourself or for your family through your employer, check out your coverage options on your state's Marketplace. Familiarize yourself with the new protections guaranteed to you and your spouse or partner; you can start by reading Chapter 1 of this book. If you have questions about how the ACA impacts your specific household situation, contact a customer service representative at Healthcare.gov by visiting the website and clicking on "Live Chat," or by calling 800-318-2596 (or 855-889-4325 for TTY users).

Assisting the Self-Employed

Anyone who is self-employed can now use the Marketplace to search for health insurance plan options and to sign up for coverage. The ACA offers significant potential benefits for self-employed people by promoting a robust Marketplace in which insurers offer more competitive rates to individuals than they offered in the past.

In addition, all the ACA rights and protections that we outline in Chapter 1 apply to every insurance plan offered on the Marketplace. Therefore, if you're self-employed and you're shopping for coverage on your state's Marketplace website, you can rest assured that the following is true:

- You cannot be denied coverage just because you have a preexisting condition.
- You cannot be charged a higher premium if you're a woman.
- You won't lose your coverage just because you become seriously ill and your medical bills escalate.

✔ Your insurance company cannot raise your premium rates astronomically from one year to the next unless it can demonstrate why doing so is justified.

✔ If you face a serious health crisis, your out-of-pocket costs in a given year are capped at a maximum set by the federal government.

✔ The insurance company cannot set an annual or lifetime maximum benefit limit, so your covered benefits will never run out.

See Chapter 1 for details about these protections and additional considerations that change the healthcare landscape substantially for many self-employed workers and other people who have relied on individual coverage in the past.

Another benefit for self-employed workers is greater ease of comparison among health insurance plans. As we explain in detail in Chapter 2, the ACA requires that every insurer offering plans on the Marketplace provide a Summary of Benefits and Coverage (SBC) for each plan. The federal government designed a template for the SBC that insurers must follow so that you see the same types of information presented for each plan, making comparisons more straightforward. If you're self-employed and you've struggled in the past to make sense of your healthcare options, this apples-to-apples comparison likely will decrease confusion and simplify your decision-making process.

How do you know if you're self-employed or a small business owner? For the purposes of the ACA, if you're the only employee of your business, you're self-employed. Even if you hire independent contractors to work for you, as long as you don't have a single employee on your payroll, you're self-employed.

However, if you report income to the IRS for one or more workers, you're a small business owner because you have employees. If that's the case for you, turn to Chapter 6 for guidance on using the new SHOP Marketplace to find coverage for yourself and/or your employees. In that chapter, you also find out about tax credits you may be eligible for as a small business owner.

Covering Part-time Employees

Many part-time employees work for small businesses and aren't offered the option of getting healthcare coverage through their employers. If that's your circumstance, you're now able to search for coverage options through the Marketplace, which we explain in detail in Chapter 2. Just as you would if you were self-employed (see the preceding section), you stand to benefit from cost savings in a robust, competitive Marketplace, and you receive significant protections that guarantee your coverage won't be denied, dropped, or significantly altered even if you require substantial medical care.

Depending on your household income, you may qualify for federal subsidies in the form of tax credits that apply directly to your monthly insurance premium payments (see Chapter 4). In addition, you can find out on the Marketplace whether you or your children qualify for your state's Medicaid or CHIP program, which then means that you aren't required to purchase individual insurance coverage.

If your employer _does_ extend a healthcare coverage option to you as a part-time employee, you may not be required to take it. However, as long as your employer's plan is deemed affordable (meaning it doesn't cost you more than 9.5 percent of your household income), and as long as it offers you an acceptable amount of coverage (meaning it covers at least 60 percent of the costs of covered health services), you aren't eligible for any subsidy support on the Marketplace. Depending on whether your income qualifies you for a tax credit, your Marketplace premiums may be higher than if your employer didn't offer you an affordable and acceptable coverage option.

Helping the Unemployed

If you're currently unemployed or you become unemployed in the future, check first to find out whether your household income now qualifies you to enroll in your state's Medicaid program or CHIP. If so, you don't need to purchase any additional health coverage to comply with the ACA.

The easiest way to determine whether you qualify for Medicaid or CHIP is to submit an application on your state's Marketplace. If you and your family don't qualify for these programs, you can then immediately check the Marketplace for plan options in your state and to determine whether you qualify for a tax credit that can apply directly to your insurance premium (see Chapter 4). The credit is determined based only on your household income and size; your employment status doesn't factor in. Keep in mind that any unemployment insurance payments you receive from the state count toward your household income.

When you apply on the Marketplace, you must report your current household income and also estimate your income for the next year. Doing so can be tricky when you're unemployed because your income status could change once you secure new employment. Make the most accurate estimates you can, based on your current circumstance, and ask for help from a Healthcare.gov customer service representative (by calling 800-318-2596, or 855-889-4325 for TTY users) if you get stuck.

If when enrolling in the Marketplace you provide a true estimate of your income that qualifies you for an insurance premium tax credit, and your income changes at some point during the year because you secure a new job, you want to log back into the Marketplace and update your income information. By doing so, you alert the Marketplace to the need to adjust your tax credit downward (or possibly eliminate it completely). That way, you avoid owing a tax credit reimbursement at tax time the following year.

While on the Marketplace, you can also determine whether you are exempt from needing to purchase health insurance because of your income status. Depending on your financial circumstances, you may qualify for a temporary hardship exemption, which means the federal government can't charge you a fine for not having health coverage during the period of your unemployment. This exemption would come into play if you are uninsured for less than three months out of the year. If your period of unemployment extends longer than three months, the hardship exemption might also apply if the least expensive insurance plan you can purchase would cost more than 8 percent of your household income, or if your annual income will be so low that you aren't required to file a federal tax return.

Helping with Pregnancy and Newborn Care

Before the passage of the ACA, healthcare plans weren't all required to offer maternity or newborn care. Some parents-to-be got an unpleasant surprise when they discovered that their policies, which had previously seemed quite thorough, didn't cover maternity care.

Individual health plans, in particular, rarely offered maternity coverage. And if they did, the plan premiums were often extremely high, to mitigate insurers' cost risks.

All new individual insurance plans, including those offered in the Marketplace, must offer maternity and newborn care. Medicaid offers this care, as well. Private insurers must cover certain essential health benefits at no cost to you, including the following:

- ✔ Breastfeeding support services
- ✔ Folic acid supplements
- ✔ Key prenatal screenings
- ✔ Prenatal doctor visits
- ✔ Support for the mother to stop using tobacco

Insurers must provide coverage for childbirth (although not at zero cost to the insured). And plans must provide for newborn care, including essential benefits that insurers must offer at no cost to you, such as recommended vaccines and screenings. See Chapter 3 for a rundown of the pediatric care benefits the ACA guarantees, including benefits that are guaranteed to newborns.

Here's another important point to keep in mind: Pregnancy falls into the category of *preexisting condition,* but because of the ACA, insurers can no longer deny you coverage because of it. In other words, if you're pregnant during an *enrollment period* — a time when you're eligible to sign up for new health coverage (see Chapter 2) — an insurer cannot refuse your application because you're pregnant. The insurer also cannot charge you a higher premium because of the pregnancy — or because you're a woman, for that matter. Both scenarios would have been common before the passage of the ACA but are no longer legal. (Insurers now cannot deny coverage to anyone and can raise premium costs based on only four factors, none of which includes health status or gender; see Chapter 1.)

If you're pregnant and you don't yet have health insurance coverage, don't waste any time. Take full advantage of the benefits available to you through the ACA. Sign up on your state's Marketplace website to determine whether you're eligible for coverage with Medicaid or CHIP, both of which support pregnant women (and their children) whose income is below a specific threshold. If you don't qualify for these programs, search for a Marketplace plan that fits your financial needs. Take full advantage of the prenatal care available to you so that you and your child can achieve maximum health during pregnancy and after the birth.

Finally, keep in mind that if you have health coverage but you want to change plans, pregnancy itself does not trigger a special enrollment period (see Chapter 2). If you aren't currently in an open enrollment period, you must wait either until you reach open enrollment or until your child is born. The birth of a child *does* trigger a special enrollment period, which then allows you to switch coverage, if you choose.

Part III
The Part of Tens

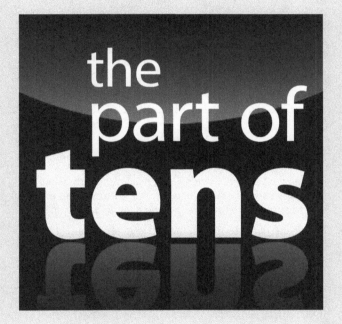

In addition to the quick bites of information you find in this part's chapters, check out ten things you really need to know about healthcare law, at www.dummies.com/extras/affordablecareact.

In this part . . .

✔ Get succinct answers to ten of the most frequently asked questions about the ACA's impact, from who needs to enroll for coverage to where to get help if you can't afford a plan.

✔ Know your rights by getting familiar with ten essential benefits the ACA provides, including preventive care, mental health services, and maternity and newborn care.

Chapter 8

Ten Frequently Asked Questions about the ACA

● ●

In This Chapter

▶ Addressing enrollment concerns

▶ Focusing on finances

▶ Getting familiar with benefits

● ●

*A*lmost everyone has questions about the Affordable Care
Act — lots of questions.

This entire book is designed to help you better understand
the benefits and protections within the law for people who
have coverage or are looking for coverage, but this chapter
gives you quick-and-easy answers to some of the questions
we hear most often. We don't offer the nitty-gritty details here,
but we hope that our responses can help set your mind at
ease about some areas of particular concern.

Who Needs to Enroll?

First, let's be clear that the majority of Americans — 85 percent —
don't need to enroll in new health insurance plans. Many
people already have private insurance coverage, such as a
group health plan sponsored by an employer, the military, or,
in some cases, an individual plan. Other people have public
insurance coverage through programs such as Medicare,
Medicaid, and the Children's Health Insurance Program
(CHIP). If you're already covered by an insurance plan, you
don't need to visit the Health Insurance Marketplace to go
shopping for a new plan (although that Marketplace is open to
everyone, so you're welcome to peruse your options).

Second, certain groups of people have been declared exempt from the ACA's provision that requires people to enroll in a healthcare plan. The exemptions apply to people who have a very low income, people who have experienced a gap in insurance coverage of less than three months, and more. We offer the complete list of exemptions in Chapter 4.

If you don't have healthcare insurance and you aren't part of an exempt group, you must enroll for coverage or you will pay a tax penalty and be responsible for all your medical bills. In that case, you need to get familiar with the Marketplace and determine when you're able to enroll (during either open enrollment or a special enrollment period; we explain both in the upcoming section "When Can I Enroll?").

Can I Enroll in a Marketplace Plan If I Already Have Insurance?

Nearly all people can shop the plan options on their state's Health Insurance Marketplace and enroll in one of the offered plans, if desired. That's the short answer, and here's the longer version:

If you have coverage through your employer, and if the plan your employer provides is deemed to be affordable and to provide what's called *minimum value,* you may not qualify on the Marketplace for discounts, or subsidies, on insurance premiums and out-of-pocket costs, no matter what your income is. To clarify, your employer's plan is considered affordable if your premium costs for the lowest-cost plan (for just you, not including family members) amount to less than 9.5 percent of your annual household income. That plan has minimum value if it pays for at least 60 percent of the costs of covered healthcare services. And if your job plan meets these criteria, you may not qualify for savings on Marketplace plans that another person at your income level might qualify for.

When in doubt, do some research. Go to your state's Marketplace website (which you can find by starting at www.healthcare.gov/what-is-the-marketplace-in-my-state), and find out what's available to you and how much it costs. You're under no obligation to purchase coverage, and it's better to know your options than to make assumptions.

When Can I Enroll?

In 2013, when the Health Insurance Marketplace websites first went live, we had our first experience with *open enrollment,* a period of time during which anyone who needs coverage or wants to switch policies can do so. That first open enrollment period was slated to last six months because so many people needed to sign up for insurance for the first time.

Starting in 2014, the rules are slightly different. The Marketplace sites will still have an annual open enrollment period for signing up and for purchasing coverage the following year. That period will last two months — from November 15 to January 15 — for coverage that begins in 2015. Check for open enrollment periods for 2016 and beyond.

You can enroll at other times of the year if you experience a *qualifying life event.* If you lose your job and, therefore, lose your insurance coverage, for example, you have 60 days to shop for a new plan on the Marketplace. The same is true if you get married or divorced, your spouse dies, you have a baby, you move and lose your insurance, or you experience another life-changing event covered by the ACA. In these cases, you're granted a special enrollment period that doesn't exist for the general public. Otherwise, if you're already insured and just looking to switch to another plan, you must wait for an open enrollment period.

How Much Am I Going to Have to Pay for Insurance?

If you already have a plan you purchased individually or one your employer offers, you likely won't see a significant change in the cost of your premium. However, you may find that premiums do change for these reasons:

✔ **Your plan coverage increases:** Some insurers may raise plan premiums to reflect an increase in the quality and scope of your coverage. As we explain in Chapter 3, many plans are now required to provide essential health benefits as defined by the ACA. This requirement expands some plans' coverage. If you're in this situation, you have two options:

- *Compare out-of-pocket costs:* Get familiar enough with your new plan coverage to determine how much you likely will save in out-of-pocket costs for using healthcare services each year. For example, you'll pay nothing out of pocket for recommended vaccinations. Estimate your savings and see if they weigh favorably against the premium increase.

- *Go shopping on the Marketplace:* If your current plan changes or your insurer switches your plan to comply with the ACA, you can shop for a new plan on your state's Health Insurance Marketplace and still potentially qualify for savings based on your annual income.

✔ **Plan competition may increase:** Depending on the state you live in, you may see a decrease in your premiums because your insurer must compete with plans offered via the Health Insurance Marketplace. If your state has a robust Marketplace with many plan options to choose from, your current insurer may need to reduce premiums to remain competitive.

For the uninsured, the amount you need to spend to comply with the ACA's individual mandate depends largely on your household income. Low-income households may be exempt from needing to get insurance coverage, depending on what your state offers for Medicaid inclusion and for plan options on the Marketplace. Individuals and households with higher incomes may still qualify for reduced costs for purchasing a plan through the Marketplace. Check out www.healthcare.gov/will-i-qualify-to-save-on-monthly-premiums to see income ranges that may qualify for plan savings, depending on the number of people in your household.

In general, someone who is uninsured, who isn't exempt from needing coverage, and who qualifies for financial help can expect to pay between 2 and 9.5 percent of his income to purchase a plan, depending on the income level and on the plan selected. See Chapter 4 for a discussion of costs and financial assistance. You have different plan categories to choose from, which greatly affects your premium costs versus out-of-pocket costs; see Chapter 3 for the scoop on available plan categories.

What If I Can't Afford to Buy Health Insurance?

Under the ACA, certain people who meet a certain threshold won't face tax penalties if they don't have insurance. For example, if you aren't required to file a federal tax return because your income is too low, you are exempt from needing to purchase coverage.

As part of the ACA, states have the option to expand their Medicaid program. Many (though not all) states have expanded their Medicaid program to provide insurance coverage to larger numbers of low-income individuals. But if you don't qualify for Medicaid in your state, and if the lowest premium cost available on your state's Marketplace equals more than 8 percent of your household income, you may be exempt from needing to purchase coverage.

Why do we say *may*? Because unless your income is low enough that you don't need to file a tax return, you can't simply assume that you qualify for an exemption. You must apply for that exemption either when filing your federal income taxes or by visiting your state's Health Insurance Marketplace. And you need to do so proactively; don't wait until you've been assessed a fee for noncompliance with the ACA (which we discuss in the next section).

What Happens If I Don't Sign Up?

If you aren't exempt under the ACA and can afford to purchase insurance and you choose not to, you may face financial penalties in two forms:

  ✔ **A tax penalty:** You pay the higher of two amounts:

 • A percentage of your annual household income, which starts at 1 percent in 2014 and increases each year. (By 2016, for example, the fee is assessed at 2.5 percent of your annual income.) This amount is capped at a certain amount, which we detail in Chapter 4.

- A flat rate, assessed on a monthly basis, which also increases each year. In 2014, this fee amounts to $95 per person, per year, and $47.50 per child under 18, per year. Per family, the 2014 cap is $285 per year. (You pay according to the number of months you're without coverage during the year.)

✔ **Healthcare expenses:** If you incur medical expenses while you don't have coverage, you must pay 100 percent of those expenses. If you don't or can't pay them, you face the full consequences of not paying, up to and including bankruptcy.

Even if you pay a tax penalty for lack of coverage, you still don't have insurance, so you face paying 100 percent of your medical expenses.

Can I Choose My Own Doctors?

The ACA requires that all people purchasing new plan coverage through the Marketplace or through a new group plan be able to choose their own primary care doctor from the list of network providers.

Check the list of participating providers to see if your regular doctor participates in the plan.

If you have coverage through a *grandfathered* plan, which we explain in Chapter 1, that plan isn't required to let you select your own primary care doctor. (It *may* allow you to do so, but it isn't required to do so.) If your plan is grandfathered, your insurance company must clearly state that fact in information it provides you about your coverage.

Can I Switch Plans?

This question can be asked in a number of circumstances:

✔ *If you have job-based insurance that changes because of the ACA,* you have the option to shop on the Health Insurance Marketplace for a new plan during the open enrollment period, just like anyone else shopping for a new plan. However, you won't qualify for financial assistance unless your employer's plan doesn't meet the ACA criteria for affordability and value, as we explain in the earlier section "Can I Enroll in a Marketplace Plan If I Already Have Insurance?"

✔ *If you have private individual insurance not through your job or Medicare or Medicaid,* you have the right to shop for a new plan on the Marketplace. Check with your current insurer to find out whether you need to wait until the end of your policy year before doing so. Your insurance company can verify whether you need to work with the Marketplace during the open enrollment period or whether you qualify to take advantage of a special enrollment period when your plan is ending.

✔ *If you purchase a plan through the Marketplace and decide that another plan is better,* you can switch plans during the next open enrollment period. If you select a plan during open enrollment and change your mind quickly — before your coverage begins — you can change your plan before its start date (as long as you're still in the open enrollment period).

Do My Medicare Benefits Change?

The ACA improves Medicare benefits by covering more preventive benefits and reducing the costs of prescription drugs.

For example, if you have Medicare, you can work with your doctor on a prevention plan to keep you as healthy as possible. As we detail in Chapter 5, per the ACA, you are entitled to the following preventive benefits at no cost to you:

✔ A yearly wellness visit.

✔ Screenings to prevent and detect health problems, including screenings for diabetes, high cholesterol, and certain cancers. Mammograms and colonoscopies, for example, are covered at no cost to you.

✔ Recommended vaccines to help prevent health problems.

If you have Medicare Part D and fall into the prescription drug coverage gap (the *doughnut hole*), because of the ACA, you now receive significant discounts on many brand-name and generic prescription drugs. The ACA provides that the Part D discounts will gradually increase until 2020, when the doughnut hole will disappear. However, everyone with Medicare Part D will still have out-of-pocket costs for premiums and copayments, just like you do now before you reach the doughnut hole. You will still be responsible for paying your premiums and deductible as well as 25 percent of your prescription drug costs until you reach catastrophic coverage. For details, see Chapter 5.

What If I Have a Chronic Illness or a History of Disease?

One aspect of the ACA that many people have really latched onto is the provision that prohibits insurance companies from dropping coverage for, denying coverage to, or raising rates for people just because they have less-than-perfect health history.

Before the ACA, if you were diagnosed with cancer, diabetes, or a heart condition, for example, you weren't guaranteed that your insurer would continue to provide coverage. And if it did continue coverage, you might have seen your rates climb each successive year. After all, the insurance company runs higher financial risks if it covers someone who is very likely to require significant medical treatment.

Likewise, an uninsured person with a chronic illness or history of disease would very likely have been denied coverage by any insurance plan applied to. Again, before the ACA, that treatment was legal.

But the ACA provides for what's called *guaranteed issue:* An insurer cannot deny you coverage, including for preexisting conditions. And if you already have insurance, your insurer cannot drop your coverage if you get sick or raise your premiums just because of your health condition. As we explain in Chapter 1, an insurer can consider only four factors when setting or changing your premiums, and none relates to your health.

Chapter 9

Ten Essential Benefits of the ACA

*T*he ACA requires that all new health plans sold on the Health Insurance Marketplace and offered to people who buy health insurance on their own or in small groups include, at a minimum, a set of essential health benefits. We describe them in this chapter, and you can find more information on this topic in Chapter 3. These essential benefits are important because they provide people with a standard set of comprehensive benefits and because they offer a way to compare plans on an apples-to-apples basis.

Before the ACA, less than 2 percent of individual health plans provided all ten of the essential benefits covered in this chapter, according to one study. Read on to learn exactly what these essential benefits are.

Ambulatory Patient Services

Often called *outpatient* care, ambulatory patient services are the most common form of health care you get without being admitted to a hospital. Nearly all health insurance plans already provided this coverage. Details about the plans' networks and access to doctors vary, but the law says the networks' size must be "sufficient."

Prescription Drugs

Many plans used to offer prescription drug coverage only as an option at extra cost. But under the ACA, all individual and small-group plans will cover at least one drug in every category and class in the *U.S. Pharmacopeia,* an official publication of approved medications in this country. Prescription drug costs also count toward out-of-pocket caps on medical expenses.

Emergency Care

Imagine that you go to a hospital emergency room with a sudden and serious condition, such as the symptoms of a heart attack or stroke. Most plans already covered the emergency visit. But under the ACA, emergency room visits for urgent care don't require preauthorization, and your benefits need to be the same for an in- and out-of-network emergency room visit.

Mental Health Services

Many insurance plans didn't previously cover mental or behavioral health services, but that has changed under the law. In some states, coverage may be limited to a set number of therapy visits per year.

Hospitalization

Under the ACA, your insurer must cover your hospitalization, although you may have to pay 20 percent of the bill or more if you haven't reached your out-of-pocket limit. Some hospitals charge $2,000 a day for room and board alone, and $20,000 with medical services, so those bills can soar. Before the ACA, medical costs helped bankrupt hundreds of thousands of American households per year — including many who thought they had decent insurance until they were diagnosed with a serious illness.

Rehabilitative and Habilitative Services

Before the ACA, if you were injured or became ill, your insurance may have covered rehabilitation therapies to help you regain your ability to speak, walk, or work. Plans often covered medical equipment, too, including canes, knee braces, walkers, and wheelchairs. Few plans, however, addressed the ACA's essential requirement for "habilitative" services, which are therapies to help overcome long-term disabilities, such as help that accompanies a disease like multiple sclerosis or disabilities from developmental delays.

Preventive and Wellness Services

Many experts believe this benefit could help rein in the nation's rising medical costs. The idea is to get people to see doctors, sometimes at no cost to you, and make healthier choices before they get sick and run up medical bills. For example, if you have Medicare, you're allowed a free annual wellness visit with your doctor to discuss your health. Check out Chapter 3 for details on preventive and wellness services covered by the ACA.

Laboratory Services

The ACA codifies the full set of preventive screening tests — including prostate exams and Pap smears — that individual and small-group insurers must cover, but you can still be billed for "diagnostic" tests that doctors order when you have symptoms of disease. Costs can range from $20 for a lab test to 30 percent of a magnetic resonance imaging scan (MRI).

Pediatric Dental and Vision Care

Under the law, children under age 19 are able to get comprehensive dental and vision care, although the minimum benefit varies from state to state. For example, some plans may allow children to have their teeth cleaned twice a year, as well as receive X-rays, fillings, and medically necessary orthodontia. In addition, children under age 19 may get an eye exam and one pair of glasses or set of contact lenses a year. Relatively few health plans previously covered children's dental or vision services.

Maternity and Newborn Care

The ACA classifies prenatal care as a preventive service that must be provided at no extra cost. It also requires insurers to cover childbirth, as well as the newborn infant's care. These maternity benefits are a welcome breakthrough; two-thirds of individual plans traditionally excluded this type of coverage.

Appendix

Resources for More Information about the ACA

*W*e don't pretend to have addressed every issue of the Affordable Care Act (ACA) in this short book. For this reason, we encourage you to use online resources such as the ones listed here to learn more.

 If you don't have a computer or you prefer talking to a person, we provide phone numbers where applicable.

AARP Resources

AARP has created an online tool at www.HealthLawAnswers. org that is easy to use and provides personalized information for you, based on your answers to a few simple questions. The tool takes only a few minutes to complete. At the end, you will receive a report with information about what the health care law means for you and your family. The tool will also provide you with resources in your area to get additional information and assistance.

This same tool is available in Spanish at www.mileyde salud.org.

Visit any of these AARP links for more information about the healthcare law:

- To get a refresher on ACA basics, including how it affects families, small businesses, people who have Medicare, and more, read AARP's Health Law Facts at www.HealthLawFacts.org or in Spanish at www.LeydeSalud.org.

- ✔ Visit The Health Care Law: More Choices, More Protections (http://healthlawanswers.aarp.org/node/335) for a quick overview of the ACA's key provisions.

- ✔ Check out Choosing a Health Care Plan: Coverage, Cost, Compare (http://healthlawanswers.aarp.org/node/334) for tips on how to shop smartly if you're in the market for new health coverage.

- ✔ If you own a small business, head to What the Health Care Law Means for Small Businesses (http://healthlawanswers.aarp.org/node/824).

- ✔ If you work for a small business, you may find the information at What the Health Care Law Means for Employees of Small Businesses (http://healthlawanswers.aarp.org/node/333) helpful.

AARP's website offers a variety of information about the ACA and will be updated on an ongoing basis so you're kept in the loop. Visit www.aarp.org at any time, and click on the "Health" tab. From there, click on the "Health Insurance" tab, and you'll find the full array of tools and information we've created to serve you.

Government Resources

If you don't have a computer or simply feel more comfortable talking with a real, live human to get the information you need, you can call the Health Insurance Marketplace toll-free at 800-318-2596 any time of day, seven days a week, in 150 languages. (If you use TTY, call 855-889-4325.) The customer service representatives who answer these calls can help you get your questions answered and get information about the Marketplace in your state.

You can also find a wealth of information online. Here we mention some of the key tools that federal government agencies have established to help you get the coverage you need and find answers to your insurance questions.

Health Insurance Marketplace

At www.HealthCare.gov, or www.CuidadoDeSalud.gov for Spanish, you can shop for and compare health plans.

Representatives can answer your questions in 150 languages. This website is updated regularly so you can get key information about enrollment period deadlines and other items you may need to act on.

No one is required to visit www.HealthCare.gov to secure health insurance coverage. If you don't currently have coverage, you can use an insurance agent or broker to purchase a plan. However, this government website is the only place to go if your income qualifies you for a subsidy to offset part of your insurance premiums (see Chapter 4). If you suspect that you may qualify for your state's Medicaid program or Children's Health Insurance Program (CHIP), which we explain in Chapter 1, you also want to start with www.HealthCare.gov to find out for certain. If you have any doubt about whether you may qualify for federal assistance or state insurance coverage, definitely apply through this website to determine your eligibility. You don't want to risk not having coverage, and you don't want to leave any government support lying on the table.

Medicaid

If your income is low, you can get your questions about Medicaid eligibility answered in the Health Insurance Marketplace or by visiting www.Medicaid.gov. To research information about the Medicaid program in your home state, you can use this link: medicaid.gov/Medicaid-CHIP-Program-Information/ By-State/By-State.html. You can also find direct links and phone numbers to state Medicaid programs at www. HealthLawAnswers.org.

TRICARE and veterans' benefits

If you're an active or retired service member or a family member of someone who is, visit www.tricare.mil to get your TRICARE and veterans' benefits questions answered. To get contact information for support in the area where you live or are stationed, use this link: www.tricare.mil/ ContactUs/CallUs.aspx.

U.S. military veterans can also find support from the U.S. Department of Veterans Affairs by calling 800-827-1000 or visiting www.va.gov.

Medicare

If you are (or soon will be) over the age of 65, you don't use the Health Insurance Marketplace to find answers about your Medicare coverage. (Medicare is also available to some younger people who have long-term disabilities.)

If you have questions about your Medicare eligibility or coverage, call 800-633-4227 or visit www.Medicare.gov.

In addition, people who qualify for Medicare (and their family members) can find support through the federally funded State Health Insurance Assistance Program (SHIP). This support takes the form of individual health insurance counseling, either by phone or in person, as well as access to public education and information programs. To find the SHIP office in your state, call 800-677-1116 or visit www.SHIPtalk.org.

Small Business Health Options Program (SHOP)

Small business owners can find information tailored to their concerns and needs by visiting www.HealthCare.gov and selecting the "Small Businesses" tab to locate details about the Small Business Health Options Program (SHOP). They can also call the Health Insurance Marketplace at 800-218-2596 to speak with a customer service representative.

In addition, the U.S. Small Business Administration (SBA) has a rich history of providing a broad spectrum of support to small businesses. Visit www.sba.gov.healthcare or call 800-827-5722.

Index

Notes

Notes

Notes

Notes

Notes

Notes

Notes

Notes

Notes

Notes

Notes

About the Authors

As Advisor of AARP's Education and Outreach team, **Lisa Yagoda** serves as issue expert for educating AARP members and the public on the Affordable Care Act, Medicare, health care coverage, and health quality. Prior to her arrival at AARP, Lisa served as Senior Policy Associate for Aging at the National Association of Social Workers (NASW), where she was responsible for policy development on issues that impact both professionals in the aging field and older consumers. Lisa was a former Eldercare Consultant to FannieMae, where she established the first private-public partnership of its kind designed to help employees with eldercare concerns at their work site. Lisa began her career serving older adults at a local Area Agency on Aging, as manager of a fee-for-service case management and counseling program for older adults and their families. She has served on several advisory panels focused on Medicare, health, and long-term care. Lisa holds a Master's degree in Social Work from the National Catholic School of Social Service. She is a licensed clinical social worker in the District of Columbia.

As Vice President of Health for AARP's Education and Outreach group, **Nicole Duritz** leads AARP's public education efforts on a variety of issues, including health security, Medicare, and the Affordable Care Act. In this role, Nicole manages a team that develops and designs consumer-focused resources and tools to ensure that the 50+ population has the information and support necessary to make decisions on critical life issues. Prior to her work in Education and Outreach, Nicole served as Campaign Director for AARP's Health Implementation Campaign and was responsible for developing and driving the execution of the campaign strategy. Nicole's tenure with AARP spans more than 18 years, including work on strategic policy planning, voter education, and Internet advocacy. Prior to joining AARP, Nicole was a principal with e-advocates, a multi-million dollar internet advocacy consulting firm. She started her career working for the U.S. House of Representatives Energy and Commerce Subcommittee on Health and the Environment.

Joan Friedman is a writer and editor who works at Cornell University. She has worked on more than 80 books *For Dummies* on subjects related to finance, education, religion, health, and more.

Authors' Acknowledgments

In recognition of their contributions to this book, the authors would like to thank AARP experts Patricia Barry, Joyce Dubow, Lynda Flowers, Harriet Komisar, Keith Lind, Leigh Purvis, Michael Schuster, Geraldine Smolka, and Lina Walker; AARP Director of Books Jodi Lipson; Wiley editors Stacy Kennedy, Linda Brandon, and Krista Hansing; and technical editor JoAnn Volk.

Publisher's Acknowledgments

Acquisitions Editor: Stacy Kennedy

Project Editor: Linda Brandon

Copy Editor: Krista Hansing

Technical Editor: JoAnn C. Volk

Art Coordinator: Alicia B. South

Project Coordinator: Rebekah Brownson

Cover Photos: ©iStockphoto.com/tetmc

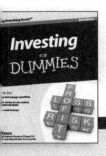 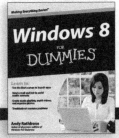 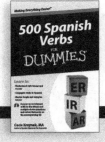 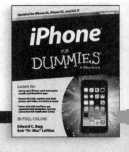

Math & Science

Algebra I For Dummies,
2nd Edition
978-0-470-55964-2

Anatomy and Physiology
For Dummies, 2nd Edition
978-0-470-92326-9

Astronomy For Dummies,
3rd Edition
978-1-118-37697-3

Biology For Dummies,
2nd Edition
978-0-470-59875-7

Chemistry For Dummies,
2nd Edition
978-1-118-00730-3

1001 Algebra II Practice
Problems For Dummies
978-1-118-44662-1

Microsoft Office

Excel 2013 For Dummies
978-1-118-51012-4

Office 2013 All-in-One
For Dummies
978-1-118-51636-2

PowerPoint 2013 For Dummies
978-1-118-50253-2

Word 2013 For Dummies
978-1-118-49123-2

Music

Blues Harmonica For Dummies
978-1-118-25269-7

Guitar For Dummies, 3rd Edition
978-1-118-11554-1

iPod & iTunes For Dummies,
10th Edition
978-1-118-50864-0

Programming

Beginning Programming with C
For Dummies
978-1-118-73763-7

Excel VBA Programming
For Dummies, 3rd Edition
978-1-118-49037-2

Java For Dummies, 6th Edition
978-1-118-40780-6

Religion & Inspiration

The Bible For Dummies
978-0-7645-5296-0

Buddhism For Dummies,
2nd Edition
978-1-118-02379-2

Catholicism For Dummies,
2nd Edition
978-1-118-07778-8

Self-Help & Relationships

Beating Sugar Addiction
For Dummies
978-1-118-54645-1

Meditation For Dummies,
3rd Edition
978-1-118-29144-3

Seniors

Laptops For Seniors
For Dummies, 3rd Edition
978-1-118-71105-7

Computers For Seniors
For Dummies, 3rd Edition
978-1-118-11553-4

iPad For Seniors For Dummies,
6th Edition
978-1-118-72826-0

Social Security For Dummies
978-1-118-20573-0

Smartphones & Tablets

Android Phones For Dummies,
2nd Edition
978-1-118-72030-1

Nexus Tablets For Dummies
978-1-118-77243-0

Samsung Galaxy S 4
For Dummies
978-1-118-64222-1

Samsung Galaxy Tabs
For Dummies
978-1-118-77294-2

Test Prep

ACT For Dummies, 5th Edition
978-1-118-01259-8

ASVAB For Dummies, 3rd Edition
978-0-470-63760-9

GRE For Dummies, 7th Edition
978-0-470-88921-3

Officer Candidate Tests
For Dummies
978-0-470-59876-4

Physician's Assistant Exam
For Dummies
978-1-118-11556-5

Series 7 Exam For Dummies
978-0-470-09932-2

Windows 8

Windows 8.1 All-in-One
For Dummies
978-1-118-82087-2

Windows 8.1 For Dummies
978-1-118-82121-3

Windows 8.1 For Dummies, Book
+ DVD Bundle
978-1-118-82107-7

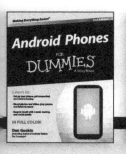
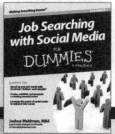
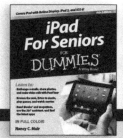
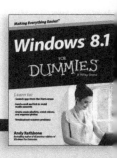

Available wherever books are sold.

For more information or to order direct visit www.dummies.com

Take Dummies with you everywhere you go!

Whether you are excited about e-books, want more from the web, must have your mobile apps, or are swept up in social media, Dummies makes everything easier.

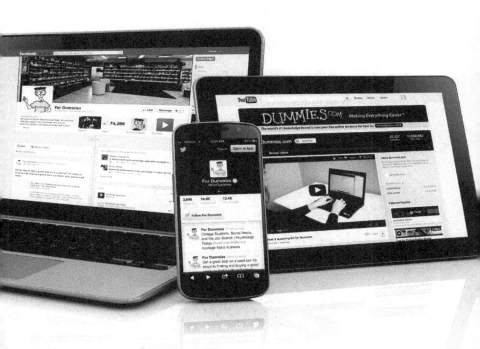

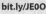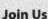

For Dummies is the global leader in the reference category and one of the most trusted and highly regarded brands in the world. No longer just focused on books, customers now have access to the For Dummies content they need in the format they want. Let us help you develop a solution that will fit your brand and help you connect with your customers.

Advertising & Sponsorships

Connect with an engaged audience on a powerful multimedia site, and position your message alongside expert how-to content.

Targeted ads · Video · Email marketing · Microsites · Sweepstakes sponsorship

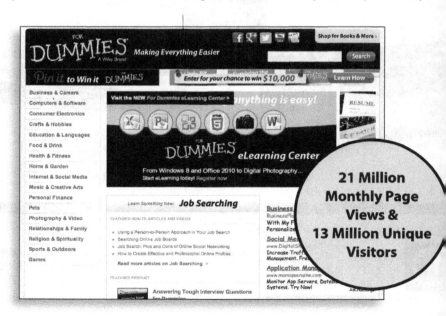

# of For Dummies

Custom Publishing

Reach a global audience in any language by creating a solution that will differentiate you from competitors, amplify your message, and encourage customers to make a buying decision.

Apps • Books • eBooks • Video • Audio • Webinars

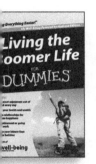 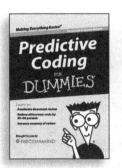 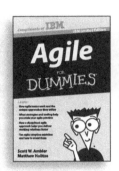 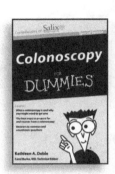

Brand Licensing & Content

Leverage the strength of the world's most popular reference brand to reach new audiences and channels of distribution.

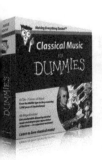 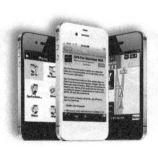 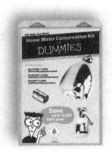 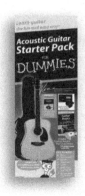

For more information, visit www.Dummies.com/biz

DUMMIES

A Wiley Brand

Dummies products make life easier!

- DIY
- Consumer Electronics
- Crafts
- Software

- Cookware
- Hobbies
- Videos

- Music
- Games
- and More!

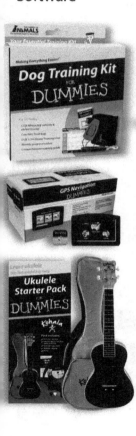

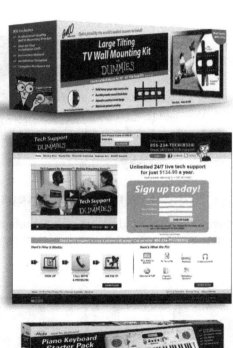

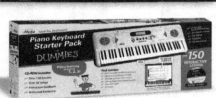

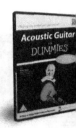

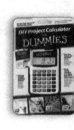

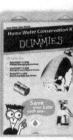

For more information, go to **Dummies.com** and search the store by category.